Tim Johansson

Telemedicine in Acute Stroke Care

Tim Johansson

Telemedicine in Acute Stroke Care

– the TESSA Model

Südwestdeutscher Verlag für Hochschulschriften

Impressum/Imprint (nur für Deutschland/only for Germany)
Bibliografische Information der Deutschen Nationalbibliothek: Die Deutsche Nationalbibliothek verzeichnet diese Publikation in der Deutschen Nationalbibliografie; detaillierte bibliografische Daten sind im Internet über http://dnb.d-nb.de abrufbar.
Alle in diesem Buch genannten Marken und Produktnamen unterliegen warenzeichen-, marken- oder patentrechtlichem Schutz bzw. sind Warenzeichen oder eingetragene Warenzeichen der jeweiligen Inhaber. Die Wiedergabe von Marken, Produktnamen, Gebrauchsnamen, Handelsnamen, Warenbezeichnungen u.s.w. in diesem Werk berechtigt auch ohne besondere Kennzeichnung nicht zu der Annahme, dass solche Namen im Sinne der Warenzeichen- und Markenschutzgesetzgebung als frei zu betrachten wären und daher von jedermann benutzt werden dürften.

Coverbild: www.ingimage.com

Verlag: Südwestdeutscher Verlag für Hochschulschriften GmbH & Co. KG
Heinrich-Böcking-Str. 6-8, 66121 Saarbrücken, Deutschland
Telefon +49 681 37 20 271-1, Telefax +49 681 37 20 271-0
Email: info@svh-verlag.de

Approved by: Salzburg, Paracelsus Medizinische Privatuniversität, Diss.,2011

Herstellung in Deutschland:
Schaltungsdienst Lange o.H.G., Berlin
Books on Demand GmbH, Norderstedt
Reha GmbH, Saarbrücken
Amazon Distribution GmbH, Leipzig
ISBN: 978-3-8381-3111-5

Imprint (only for USA, GB)
Bibliographic information published by the Deutsche Nationalbibliothek: The Deutsche Nationalbibliothek lists this publication in the Deutsche Nationalbibliografie; detailed bibliographic data are available in the Internet at http://dnb.d-nb.de.
Any brand names and product names mentioned in this book are subject to trademark, brand or patent protection and are trademarks or registered trademarks of their respective holders. The use of brand names, product names, common names, trade names, product descriptions etc. even without a particular marking in this works is in no way to be construed to mean that such names may be regarded as unrestricted in respect of trademark and brand protection legislation and could thus be used by anyone.

Cover image: www.ingimage.com

Publisher: Südwestdeutscher Verlag für Hochschulschriften GmbH & Co. KG
Heinrich-Böcking-Str. 6-8, 66121 Saarbrücken, Germany
Phone +49 681 37 20 271-1, Fax +49 681 37 20 271-0
Email: info@svh-verlag.de

Printed in the U.S.A.
Printed in the U.K. by (see last page)
ISBN: 978-3-8381-3111-5

Copyright © 2012 by the author and Südwestdeutscher Verlag für Hochschulschriften GmbH & Co. KG and licensors
All rights reserved. Saarbrücken 2012

Table of contents

1 Summary (in german) 3
2 Abstract 5
3 Introduction 7
4 Background 9
    4.1 Stroke as Diagnoses 9
    4.2 Stroke Management: Stroke Unit 9
    4.3 Access to Health Services and Citizens Stroke Education ... 9
    4.4 General Stroke Treatment and Monitoring 10
    4.5 Acute Management of Ischemic Stroke 10
    4.6 Specific Treatment: Recanalization Therapy 11
        4.6.1 Cost and Cost-Effectiveness of Intravenous Thrombolysis ... 11
    4.7 Stroke in Austria 12
    4.8 Telemedicine per Definition 14
    4.9 Telemedicine in Stroke Management 15
    4.10 Literature review: Telemedicine in Acute Stroke Care 15
        4.10.1 Telemedicine Models and Processes 16
        4.10.2 Results of Telemedicine in Acute Stroke 17
5 Method and Material 21
    5.1 Objectives and hypothesis 21
    5.2 Research Questioning 21
    5.3 Study Design, Settings and Study Population 21
    5.4 Data Collection 22
    5.5 Outcomes Measures 22
    5.6 Statistical Analysis 23
    5.7 Study Intervention: Telestroke in the county of Salzburg (TESSA) ... 24
6 Results 26
7 Discussion 36
    7.1 Methodological Discussion: 39
8 Conclusion 41
9 References 42

List of figures

Figure 3.7-1: Stroke units in Austria 14
Figure 3.9-2: Telestroke schematic illustration 17

List of tables

Tab. 3.9-1: tPA via telephone or video consultation interventions. 19
Tab. 4.7-2: TESSA Cooperating hospitals 24
Tab. 5-3: Baseline data 27
Tab. 5-4: Indicators for quality of acute stroke care 29
Tab. 5-5: Cause of death (in hospital) 30
Tab. 5-6: Distribution of regional hospital s consultations 30
Tab. 5-7. Patients neurological function: NIHSS and Rankin Scale 32
Tab. 5-8: In hospital complications 33
Tab. 5-9: Medical treatment, PTA and secondary prophylaxis 34
Tab. 5-10: Patient status and living situation at 3 months follow-up 35
Tab. 6-11: Comparisons of safety of tPA treatment (3h window) 37

1 Summary (in german)

In den industrialisierten Ländern zählt Schlaganfall zur dritthäufigsten Todesursache nach Herz-Kreislauferkrankungen und Krebs. Schlaganfall ist auch eine der häufigsten Ursachen für dauerhafte Behinderungen. Ein akuter Schlaganfall benötigt ein rasches Verfahren und eine präzise Diagnose („time is brain") um Langzeitbehinderungen zu mindern. Patienten, die in spezialisierten Schlaganfallzentren, sog. „Stroke Units" behandelt werden, haben eine bessere Überlebenschance und Gesundheitsprognose als konventionell behandelte Schlaganfallpatienten. Intravenöse Thrombolyse ist eine effektive Therapie, wenn sie innerhalb der ersten 3 Stunden nach den Schlaganfallsymptomen injiziert wird. Thrombolyse, der Tissue Plasminogen Activator (tPA) ist eine Substanz, die ein Blutgerinnsel auflösen kann und ist mit einer niedrigen Morbidität und Mortalität verbunden. Telemedizin ermöglicht es nun, dass neurologische Experten mit regionalen Ärzten, ohne Verzögerung und geografischer Barriere, kommunizieren können, und dadurch eine schnelle Betreuung der Patienten möglich wird. Die putativen Vorteile von Telemedizin sind zum einen die verbesserte Qualität des Schlaganfallmanagements und zum anderen die erhörte Rate von intravenösen Thrombolysen.

Die Zielsetzung dieser Dissertation ist die Sicherheit und Wirksamkeit von intravenöser Thrombolyse via Videokonsultation gemeinsam mit teleradiologischen verfahren gefolgt von einem Patiententransport zu einer spezialisierten Stroke Unit zu untersuchen. Die Hypothese ist das Schlaganfallpatienten, die in regionalen Krankenhäusern mit intravenösen tPA behandelt werden die gleiche Chance für einen guten Gesundheitszustand haben wie Patienten, die an einer spezialisierten Stroke Unit behandelt werden. Diese Telestroke Intervention ermöglicht den Schlaganfallpatienten den Zugang zu einer standardisierten Stroke Unit Behandlung sowie Zugang zu neurochirurgischen und Neuro-Angiographische Interventionen. Als Methode wurde eine retrospektive kontrollierte Studie durchgeführt.

Insgesamt wurden 47 Telethrombolyse Patienten in der Telemedizingruppe inkludiert während als Kontrollgruppe 304 tPA behandelte Patienten an einer spezialisierten Stroke Unit als Kontrollgruppe benutzt wurden. Die Charakteristika der Population wie Alter, Geschlecht und Risikofaktoren waren zwischen den Gruppen ähnlich. Der Beginn der Symptomatik bis zur intravenösen Thrombolyse (Onset – Lyse –Zeit) war in der Telemedizingruppe kürzer als in der Kontrollgruppe, jedoch nicht signifikant, 113 versus 122 Minuten. Die Mortalität zwischen den Gruppen zeigte keine signifikante unterschiede p=0,056). In der Telemedizingruppe wurden in 6,4% der Fälle hämorrhagische Komplikationen festgestellt, im Vergleich dazu 7,6% in der Kontrollgruppe. Laut der Epikrise wurden keine Komplikationen beim Patiententransport registriert. Bei der Entlassung hatten 38,3% der Patienten in der Telemedizingruppe einen guten Gesundheitszustand (modified Rankin Scale, dichotome Analyse 0-1) im Vergleich zu 32% in der Kontrollgruppe. Nach 3 Monate lag die Gesamtmortalität in der Telethrombolysegruppe bei 19,1% im Vergleich zu 12,5% in der Kontrollgruppe (p=0,248). 46,7% in der Telemedizingruppe hatten einen guten Gesundheitszustand und 42,5% in der Kontrollgruppe.

Telemedizinische Interventionen können das Wissen und die Expertise von spezialisierten Schlaganfallzentren zu regionalen neurologisch unterversorgten Regionen verbreiten. Effektive Behandlungstherapien wie intravenöse tPA können häufiger eingesetzt werden, was eine bessere Gesundheitsprognose für die Patienten bedeutet. Bei der Entlassung und nach 3 Monate war die Mortalität und der Gesundheitszustand der Patienten in der Telemedizingruppe und Kontrollgruppe vergleichbar. Das heißt intravnöse Thrombolyse via Telemedizin und der anschließende Patiententransport zu einer spezialisierten Stroke Unit ist sicher und wirksam.

Um die klinischen und ökonomischen Aspekte von Telestroke- Interventionen genauer analysieren zu können sind größere prospektiv kontrollierte Studien wünschenswert.

2 Abstract

Background: Stroke is the third largest cause of death after cardiovascular diseases and cancer and is a major factor of permanent disability in most industrial countries. Disparities exist in access to healthcare services due to geographical barriers and limited resources. Rural locations often lack the resources for adequate stroke management. The idea of telestroke is to transfer knowledge and expertise of acute stroke management into areas with limited neurological services.

Objective: To assess the safety and effectiveness of intravenous thrombolysis application via a real time two-way videoconferencing (VC) system combined with a teleradiological procedure followed by transfer to a specialised stroke unit.

Method: A retrospective controlled study was conducted.

Results: Between 2006 and 2009 47 stroke patients were treated via telemedicine (telethrombolysis); 304 patients treated with intravenous thrombolysis at a stroke unit served as the control group. The mean age of the patients in the telemedicine group was 66.5 years (SD ±14.4) and 71.0 years (SD ±15.5) in the control group. Mean length of stay was 6.4 (SD ±5.0) days in the telemedicine group versus 5.5 (SD ±4.6) days in the control group (p=0.255). The in-hospital mortality rate of the telemedicine group was 8.9% and 2.6% in the control group (p=0.056). Haemorrhagic bleeding occurred in 6.4% of the telemedicine group compared to 7.6% in the control group. The mean onset-to-stroke unit time was longer in the control group - 231 minutes (SD ±57.4) compared to 108 minutes (SD ±71.9) (p=0.000) in the telemedicine group. The mean onset-to-needle time was slightly shorter in the telemedicine group compared to the control group but not statistically significant, 113 minutes (SD ±39.9) versus 122 minutes (SD ±47.2) (p=0.263). No complications were reported during patient transport. At discharge from the stroke unit 38.3% of the patients in the telemedicine group had good functional outcome (mRS, dichotomized analysis 0-1) compared to 32% in the control group (p=0.506). At the 3 month follow-up, 46.7% of the patients in the telemedicine group had a good functional outcome (mRS, dichotomized analysis 0-1) versus 42.5% in the control group (p=0.694). The overall mortality at the 3 month follow-up was 19.1% in the telemedicine group and 12.5% in the control (p=0.248).

Conclusion: Health outcome at discharge and at 3 months follow-up show that telethrombolysis via VC combined by teleradiology, followed by patient transport to a stroke unit is a safe and effective form of patient management when compared to intravenous thrombolysis treatment in a specialised stroke unit. Telemedicine systems can support regional areas with insufficient neurological experience in delivering intravenous thrombolysis and so improve the quality of care and minimize inequalities in stroke care. Standardized measures to assess telestroke services would assist in the comparison between telestroke and standard care and would facilitate better comparisons across telestroke studies. More research is needed to explore the clinical and economic impact of telemedicine technologies in stroke management, so as to support policy makers in making informed decisions.

Keywords: telemedicine, acute stroke care, intravenous thrombolysis (telethrombolysis).

3 Introduction

Stroke is one of the leading causes of morbidity and mortality worldwide. In industrial countries stroke is the third largest course of death after cardiovascular diseases and cancer and a major cause of permanent disability [1]. The burden of stroke is heavy for patients and their caregivers, tax payers and society in terms of premature death, long-term disability, restricted social functioning, costs of care, lost productivity and informal caregiver time [2]. Acute stroke care requires rapid assessment, including patients medical history, neurological examination, brain imaging and expert interpretation for an accurate diagnosis. Patients who receive specialised stroke unit care are more likely to survive and make a good recovery compared to patients treated in general medical wards [3]. For acute ischemic stroke patients, intravenous thrombolysis treatment with tissue plasminogen activator (tPA) within 3 hours after the onset of stroke symptoms has been shown to reduce subsequent dependency, morbidity and mortality. tPA dissolves the obstructing blood clot, restoring blood flow before major irreversible brain damage has occurred. More recent research has also reported that intravenous tPA within 3 to 4.5 hours is effective, although the risk for intracranial haemorrhage increases [4, 5]. The problem is, however, that most stroke patients do not have access to stroke unit care and intravenous tPA, that are both primarily offered in academic stroke departments. The main reasons for this are a lack of experts (especially in nonurban areas), financial factors and delays in hospital admissions. A large number of stroke patients are unable to access a hospital with the appropriate facilities within the 3 hour treatment window for intravenous tPA [6]. In the last decade, with the development of information and communication technologies in medicine, there has been growing interest in the role that telemedicine interventions could play to improve the quality of stroke management. The primary benefit of a telemedicine system is that areas with insufficient neurological services can be supported by a stroke expert through telephone or real-time VC. Telemedicine interventions in acute stroke care may improve quality and processes in stroke care and increased use of intravenous tPA. Other putative advantages reported are reductions in costs (avoidance of patient transfer), improvements in stroke education and better efficiency in implementation of rehabilitation services [7]. This original work aims: to explore the safety and effectiveness of intravenous tPA via telemedicine and teleradiology followed by transfer to a specialised stroke unit.

For the purposes of this report the term "telestroke" is defined as: *'the process by which electronic, visual, and audio communications (including the telephone) are used to provide diagnostic and consultation support to practitioners at distant sites, assist in or directly deliver medical care to patients at distant sites and enhance the skills and knowledge of distant medical care providers'* [7].

4 Background

This chapter starts with a short introduction to stroke pathology followed by discussions of conventional stroke management with a focus on ischemic stroke. A later chapter covers stroke care in Austria. The main focus of the background chapter is reviewing the literature on telemedicine in acute stroke care.

4.1 Stroke as Diagnoses

Stroke is a sudden impairment of brain functions caused either by reduced blood flow to the brain or by a blood vessel rupturing causing hemorrhagic stroke. When ischemia happens, part of the brain cannot be supported sufficiently and brain tissue starts to die. Ischemic stroke accounts for about 80 percent and haemorrhagic stroke for about 20 percent of all cases [8].

4.2 Stroke Management: Stroke Unit

Organised stroke unit care is provided by specially trained, multidisciplinary teams that exclusively manage stroke patients. It has been shown that stroke unit care reduces mortality, morbidity and disability. Stroke units also improve different aspects of long-term quality of life and reduce length of stay in hospital [3, 9]. According to the Helsingborg Declaration 2006 on European Stroke strategies, one major goal that should be achieved by 2015 is: "All patients in Europe with stroke will have access to a continuum of care from organized stroke units in the acute phase to appropriate rehabilitation and secondary prevention measures" [10] (p. 232). Despite the strong scientific evidence for organised stroke unit care, it is still far from implemented and inequalities exist due to access issues.

4.3 Access to Health Services and Citizens Stroke Education

Non-urban environments present challenges for health care access. Normally limited access routes to health professionals exist and long travel distances to health services are common. The low population density also affects the availability of different health services. Small rural health care providers normally cannot afford equipment and personnel necessary to treat the entire array of diseases and injuries. For example, emergency care for stroke or heart attack in rural areas is associated with greater morbidity and mortality due to long transport times [11]. Stroke education for citizens is another important activity and research field. Research has shown that more than two-thirds of all stroke patients cannot be considered for intravenous thrombolytic therapy because of patient delays in seeking emergency care. Changing patients' health-care seeking behaviours when an acute stroke is suspected remains a major challenge in stroke management [10].

4.4 General Stroke Treatment and Monitoring

Once the patient has arrived in the emergency department, she or he must first be examined for potentially life threatening complications, with emphasis on airway, respiratory function and circulation. The following parameters should be monitored and/or treated in the emergency room, stroke unit or normal ward: NIHSS, electrocardiogram monitoring (first 48h of stroke onset), cardiac care, blood pressure (routine blood pressure lowering is not recommended, except for extremely elevated values >200-220/120 mmHg for ischemic stroke, >180/105 mmHg for haemorrhagic stroke), pulmonary function (oxygenation monitoring with pulse oximetry and O_2-administration in case of hypoxia, intubations), glucose metabolism (hyperglycaemia and hypoglycaemia worsens outcome), fluid and electrolytes, and body temperature (fever negatively influences outcome) [12-15].

4.5 Acute Management of Ischemic Stroke

There are six mainstays in the management of acute ischemic stroke [12-15]:
- Diagnostic measures to confirm diagnosis and provide the opportunity to make sound therapeutically decisions.
- Treatment of general conditions that influence long-term functional outcome (blood pressure, body temperature, glucose level).
- Specific therapies directed at particular aspects of stroke pathogenesis, either recanalization of a vessel occlusion or prevention of mechanisms leading to neuronal death.
- Prophylaxis and treatment of complications, either medical (such as aspiration, infections, decubital ulcers, deep venous thrombosis, or pulmonary embolism) or neurological (such as secondary haemorrhage, space-occupying oedema or seizures).
- Early secondary prevention, to reduce the incidence of early stroke recurrence.
- Early rehabilitation.

4.6 Specific Treatment: Recanalization Therapy

Administration of early thrombolytic therapy in ischemic stroke is based on the concept that early restoration of circulation in the affected brain territory by recanalization of an occluded intracranial artery preserves reversibly damaged neuronal tissue in the penumbra. The recovery of neuronal functions reduces clinical neurological disability [16]. Thrombolytic therapy is of proven benefit for selected patients with ischemic stroke. Completion of large phase III trials of intravenous thrombolytic therapy, which employed various agents, doses, and time windows, has provided a substantial database to guide clinical practice. The following recommendations have been made by centers offering thrombolysis: intravenous thrombolysis with tPA 0.9 mg/kg, maximum of 90 mg, with 10% of the dose given as a bolus, following by an infusion lasting 60 minutes) is approved in the United States and in Europe for treatment within 3 hours of onset of ischemic stroke and improves outcome significantly [17]. The sooner that tPA is given to stroke patients, the greater the benefit, especially if started within 90 min of occurrence of stroke symptoms. The benefit from the use of intravenous tPA for acute ischemic stroke beyond 3 h after onset of the symptoms is smaller, but present up to 4.5 h [4, 18]. Intravenous tPA is not recommended when the time of stroke onset cannot be ascertained reliably; this includes persons whose strokes are recognised upon awakening [15, 18]. Thrombolytic therapy is not recommended in patients with severe ischaemic stroke (NIHSS> 25), with vast early infarct signs and with extremely elevated blood pressure values because of the risk of intracranial haemorrhage. Furthermore there is a limitation of approval in patients who have any history both prior stroke and concomitant diabetes, blood glucose <2.8 or >22 mmol/l and seizure at onset of stroke [15].

4.6.1 Cost and Cost-Effectiveness of Intravenous Thrombolysis

Telemedicine seems to be a promising approach for reducing cost in stroke care, and most importantly, for reducing subsequent costs by extending the use of thrombolytic drugs. In 2003, there were an estimated 616,000 ischemic stroke cases in the United States. Demaerschalk & Todd showed in an economic analysis that over $7 million would be saved for every 2% increase in the treatment of stroke patients with intravenous thrombolysis. Between $37 and $74 million would be saved by treating 10 to 20% of ischemic stroke patients [19]. Particularly in the long-term when cost and health outcomes are considered, the use of intravenous thrombolytic therapy up to six hours after the incidence is cost-effective in terms of quality adjusted life years (QALY) gained. Treatment with tPA was associated with an additional cost of £13,581 per QALY gained during the first 12 months after treatment. When the model was run to the end of the cohort lifetime, there appeared to be a substantial cost saving of £96,565 per QALY gained [20]. Another study also showed long-term economic benefits in the use of intravenous thrombolysis. The short-term incremental cost-effectiveness ratio of intravenous thrombolysis therapy (1 year) was calculated at $55,591 US per QALY gained. In the second year the incremental cost-effectiveness ratio was $3,615 US per QALY gained. In the long term (30 years), intravenous thrombolysis treatment (tPA) is the dominant strategy compared with conservative treatment [21]. Fagan & Morgenstern showed with a Markov-model that for every 1000 patients treated with tPA (<3h), that hospitalization costs increased by $1.7 million US but rehabilitation costs decreased by $1.4 million and nursing home costs decreased by $4.8 million [22]. An economic model with the use of a hypothetical cohort of 1000 acute ischaemic stroke patients showed that tPA was saving a net cost of $3,800 (Can) per patient in the perspective of lifetime healthcare costs. The use of tPA treatment also resulted in a net benefit of 3.46 QALYs per patient [23].

4.7 Stroke in Austria

Approximately 20,000 (2.1% of the female population and 2.7% of the male population) strokes occur annually in Austria [24]. The overall mortality in Austria in 2008 was 75,083. Cerebrovascular diseases - International Classification of Diseases (ICD) codes I60-I69, were responsible for 5,358 (2,040 men and 3,318 women) deaths making it the third most numerous cause of overall mortality after cardiovascular disease and cancer [25]. 43,547 hospital discharges in 2007 were registered as cerebrovascular disease (I60-I69) [26]. Approximately one third of the Austrian population is directly or indirectly (e.g. family members) affected by stroke. Since stroke incidence increases with age [27], and Austria's population is aging and surviving longer, pressure on Austrian health services is certain to increase. The admission of stroke patients in Austria differs widely. Approximately 29% to 59% of all stroke patients are admitted in neurological wards, stroke units or stroke wards respectively. Between 13% to 33% are admitted in stroke units and between 41% to 61% are admitted in other wards [28]. 10,669 stroke patients were treated in a stroke unit in 2008 [26]. In Austria the use of intravenous thrombolytic therapy differs widely in stroke units, from no use at all to approximately 20%. On average, 3% of all ischemic stroke patients are treated with intravenous thrombolysis. It should also be noted that an infrastructure with stroke units does not guarantee a high quality of stroke care and that there is no gold standard for treatment /or/ clear system for best practice treatment available [28]. The infrastructure within Austrian stroke units also differs widely, which influences the quality and access to appropriate stroke care. The eastern parts of Austria have better stroke unit infrastructure (fig. 3.7-1). In the western parts of Austria stroke patients have limited access to stroke units. People living in southern parts in the state of Salzburg have limited access to stroke unit therapy, which is one of the main reasons for the development and implementation of the TESSA model.

Figure 1, shows the distribution of 32 stroke units in Austria in 2009 and it is clear that there is a shortage of stroke units in the western parts of Austria. One reason for this is, of course, the low population density in these areas. It is unrealistic to aim for full stroke unit coverage in lowly populated areas. In regions with lower population densities it is harder to finance and implement full coverage of stroke unit care [11, 29]. In these rural areas the use of telemedicine could be an alternative intervention/strategy to provide better stroke care [29, 30].

Figure 3.7-1: Stroke units in Austria

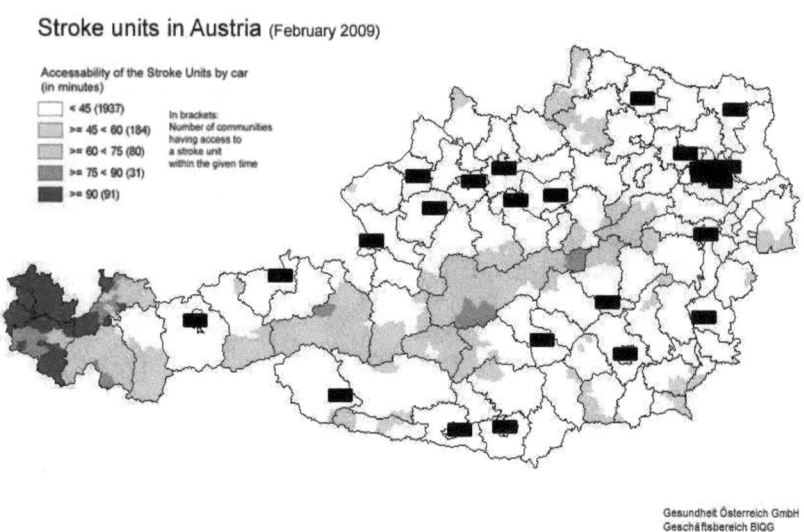

Source: Gesundheit Österreich GmbH Geschäftsbereich BIQG

4.8 Telemedicine per Definition

Telemedicine has broadly been defined as "the use of telecommunication technologies to provide medical information and services" [31](p 483). Technically, this includes all aspects of medicine practiced at a distance, such as telephone, fax, electronic mail technology, audio- and videoconferencing, transmission of still images, e-health including patient portals, remote monitoring of vital signs and nursing call centers [32, 33]. WHO define telemedicine as: "the delivery of healthcare services, where distance is a critical factor, by all healthcare professionals using information and communication technologies for the exchange of valid information for diagnosis, treatment and prevention of disease and injuries, research and evaluation, and for the continuing education of healthcare providers, all in the interests of advancing the health of individuals and their communities" [34].

4.9 Telemedicine in Stroke Management

Levine and Gorman proposed the term "telestroke" for the use of telemedicine in acute stroke intervention [35]. The primary benefit of a telemedicine system is that areas with insufficient neurological services can be supported by a stroke expert over the telephone or via a real-time VC. A telemedical stoke network can spread the knowledge and experiences from stroke units as well as increase the delivery of intravenous thrombolysis for ischemic stroke patients, which may improve the quality and processes in stroke care. Other putative advantages reported are a reduction in costs due to the avoidance of the need to transfer patients, an improvement in stroke education and improved efficiency in the implementation of rehabilitation services [7].

Telemedicine systems can offer a wider range of stroke therapies in areas with insufficient neurological facilities. Telemedicine also has a large potential to improve stroke education and quality management. Each consultation can transfer knowledge in both directions and follow-up presentations provide quality assurance [29, 30, 36, 37].

4.10 Literature review: Telemedicine in Acute Stroke Care

This literture review is based on a recently publisched systematic review on telemedicine in acute stroke care [36]. 18 studies on telemedicine technologies in acute stroke settings were included in this review. 10 of these studies used a two-way real-time audio-video conferencing system [38-47]. Three studies compared telephone consultation with video consultation [48-50] and five interventions used telephones to support community hospitals in acute stroke management [51-55]. There were two randomized controlled trials [48, 50] and one controlled clinical trial [40]. 15 studies used an observational study design such as a case series or single prospective cohorts. 13 studies reported the source of funding, with only two reporting industry funding. 15 networks with telemedical technologies in acute stroke settings were identified. 10 were located in the US, three in Germany and one each in Canada and China.

4.10.1 Telemedicine Models and Processes

There are two main approaches in the use of telemedicine technologies in acute stroke care:
- two-way real-time VC or
- a telephone consultation based support system

In a real-time VC service the neurologist can conduct a full neurological examination. The NIHSS can be determined and tPA eligibility analysed. Laboratory results and computer tomography (CT) and sometimes magnetic resonance imaging (MRI) scans can be transferred through most systems (teleradiology); otherwise these findings are verbally reported [38, 42, 43, 45, 46, 48, 51]. Based on the medical findings the stroke specialist provides the physicians with recommendations for stroke care. A two-way videoconferencing system requires monitors, video cameras and microphones located both on-site and at the stroke center. The VC networks are based either on a fixed point-to-point connection system dependent on Integrated Service Digital Network (ISDN), on a Digital Subscriber Line (DSL) or on an Internet connection. ISDN lines guarantee bandwidth availability as well as consistent service quality but restrict the accessibility of the telestroke system to the facilities where the dedicated lines are installed [43, 47]. The web-based model can be initiated from almost any location, provided that the device has access to the public Internet and the necessary software is installed. The advantage of this model is that time can be saved by avoiding the need for the consultant to travel to the hub sites which shortens the onset-to-treatment time [38, 45, 47]. When using a web-based system, the connection to a specific Internet provider may fail. Unstable bandwidths are further problems inherent to using the Internet [47].

Acute stroke patients in telemedicine programs are generally triaged by emergency physicians at community hospitals (fig. 3.9-2).

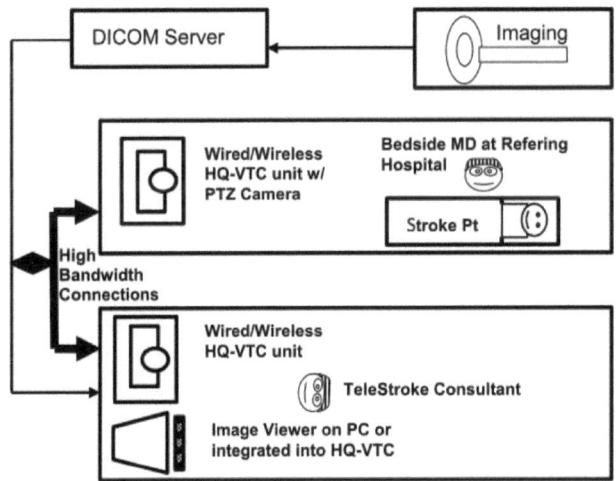

Figure 3.9-2: Telestroke schematic illustration. (Adapted from Rosenthal E, Schwamm LH. Telemedicine and stroke. In: Wootton R, Patterson V, eds. Teleneurology. London, England: Royal Society of Medicine Press, Ltd; 2005.)

Before initiating a VC the stroke center is contacted via a digital pager system or a telephone call [39, 43, 44, 47, 50]. A remote stroke expert then carries out a consultation or advises the referring physician using telemedicine technologies. In 7 studies, clinical stroke protocols were used to triage stroke patients in community hospitals [38-41, 44, 47, 51]. In most networks the stroke protocols include a guideline driven criteria list for treatment with intravenous thrombolysis [38-41, 43, 46, 51, 54].

4.10.2 Results of Telemedicine in Acute Stroke

All the telemedicine networks reported a positive experience and improved quality of care, suggesting that the implementation of such systems is feasible and acceptable. One study reported better health outcomes including reduced dependency and mortality at 3 months follow-up compared to conventional stroke care patients. The percentage of patients treated in the intervention hospitals who died within the first 3 months was 16%, compared with 18% in the control group ($p=0.20$). A total of 44% of patients in the telemedicine group had a poor outcome (mRS >3 or Barthel index <60.) after 3 months, compared with 54% in the control group ($p<0\cdot0001$) [40]. Only 3 studies reported on satisfaction with telemedicine interventions in acute stroke care. Overall, patients and health care providers reported high levels of satisfaction and acceptance, but few studies had the evaluation of satisfaction and acceptance as a main objective [42, 45, 46]. On average a VC took between 15 [39, 42] and 17.8 minutes [49]. A telephone consultation took 13.6 minutes on average [49]. Accounting for all directly related processes, such as preparation and documentation, the VC took 49.8 minutes (29–62 min) at the stroke center and 44.2 minutes (35–60 min) at the local hospital. The telephone consultation took a mean time of 27.2 minutes (15–38 min) at the stroke center and 22.3 minutes (10–29 min) at the local hospital [49].

15 studies reported on the delivery of tPA treatment via telemedicine (table 3.9-1). 9 studies used VC technologies [38-44, 46, 47], four studies were based on telephone consultations [51, 53-55] and two studies reported on the delivery of tPA via both telephone and VC technologies [45, 50]. The number of consultations differs widely between the studies, with a range of 24 to 2182 consultations. In the included studies, a total of 739 patients were treated with tPA via telemedicine. The mean age of the patients treated in the included studies ranged from 60-71 years; 45% of the patients were female. The median baseline NIHSS scores ranged from 10-14 in the telemedicine studies. The rates of intracerebral haemorrhages ranged from 0%-16.7% and the mortality rate ranged from 0-50%, although the small number of tPA treated patient in some studies strongly influence this high value. In Meyer et al. the mortality was higher in the video consultation group (39%) compared to the telephone group (12%), but after adjustment for the imbalanced NIHSS score at baseline no statistical difference was found [50].

Some studies have reported that VC methods are superior both in terms of diagnostic accuracy [48] and in terms of leading to a correct treatment decision [50], compared to telephone systems. In one study the diagnostic accuracy in the VC group was 87.7% versus 63.8% (P=0.001) in the telephone group [48]. A correct treatment decision was reported in 108 VC cases (98%), compared with 91 telephone cases (82%), (OR 10.9, 95% CI 2.7–44.6; p=0.0009) [49].

Tab. 3.9-1: tPA via telephone or video consultation interventions.

Author, Year	Consultation/No.	Receiving IV. tPA	Population Characteristic	Transported to SC	Outcomes — Mortality	Outcomes — ICH	Outcomes — Length of Stay	Outcomes — Discharge Destination	Processes (mean/min.)
Audebert, 2005 [39]	Video/ 2182	106	Mean age: 68 Female: 41% Median pre-NIHSS: 13	N/A	In-hospital 11 (10.4 %) ≤7 days, 6 (5.7%)	15 (8.5%)	12 days (median)	N/A	Door-to-needle: 76 Onset-to-hospital:65 Onset-to-needle: N/A
Audebert, 2006 [40]	Video/ N/A	80	N/A	N/A	N/A	N/A	N/A	N/A	N/A
Audebert, 2006 [41]	Video/ N/A	115	Mean age: 69.7 Female:44% Median pre-NIHSS: 12	N/A	In-hospital mortality 4 (3.5%) ≤7 days, 4 (3.5%)	9 (7.8%)	10 (median)	N/A	Door-to-needle: 68 Onset-to-hospital: 64 Onset-to-needle: 134
Choi, 2006 [43]	Video/ 328	14 (4.3%)	Mean age: 68.5 Female: 50% Median pre NIHSS 10	10 of 14 (71%) tPA patients	N/A	0	N/A	N/A	Door-to-needle: (median) 85 Onset-to-hospital: N/A Onset-to-needle: N/A
Frey, 2005 [51]	Telephone/ N/A	53	Mean age: 67.0 Female:35.8% Median pre-NIHSS: N/A	53	4 (7%)	3 (6%)	5 (1-16) (Median)	Home: 16 Rehab.: 22 Skilled nursing facility: 11	Door-to-needle: 105 Onset-to-hospital: 60 Onset-to-needle:165
Hess, 2005 [44]	Video/ 194	30 (23 %)	Mean age: 62 Female:60% Median pre-NIHSS:12.5	N/A	N/A	0	N/A	N/A	Door-to-needle: N/A Onset-to-hospital: N/A Onset-to-needle: 122
LaMonte, 2003 [45]	Video/ 27	5 (18.5%)	Mean age: N/A Female: N/A Median pre-NIHSS: N/A	5	0	0	N/A	N/A	Door-to-needle: N/A Onset-to-hospital: N/A Onset-to-needle: N/A
	Telephone/ 23	1 (4.3%)		1	0	0	N/A	N/A	
Meyer, 2008 [50]	Video/ 111	31 (28%)	Mean age: N/A Female:N/A Mean pre-NIHSS: 16.3 (video), 12.3 (telephone)	19 of 31 (61%) tPA patients	3 (12%)	2 (7%)	N/A	N/A	Door-to-needle: N/A Onset-to-hospital: N/A Onset-to-needle: N/A
	Telephone/ 111	25 (23%)		18 of 25 (72%) tPA patients	12 (39%)	2 (8%)	N/A	N/A	
Rymer, 2003 [53]	Telephone/ N/A	52	Mean age: N/A Female:N/A Median pre-NIHSS: N/A	N/A	3 (5.8%)	1 (1.9%)	N/A	N/A	Door-to-needle: N/A Onset-to-hospital: N/A Onset-to-needle: 119
Schwamm, 2004 [46]	Video/ 24	6 (25%)	Mean age: N/A Female:N/A Mean pre-NIHSS: 16.3 (8–22)	N/A	N/A	1 (16.7%)	N/A	N/A	Door-to-needle: 106 Onset-to-hospital: N/A Onset-to-needle: N/A
Vaishnav, 2008 [54]	Telephone/ N/A	123	Mean age: 64 Female: 39.8% Median pre-NIHSS: N/A	123	9 (7.5%)	14 (11.4%)	4 (mean)	Home: 47%	Door-to-needle: N/A Onset-to-hospital: 54 Onset-to-needle: 137
Waite, 2006 [38]	Video/ 88	27 (30%)	Mean age: N/A Female: N/A Median pre-NIHSS: N/A	N/A	1 (3.7%)	0	N/A	N/A	Door-to-needle: N/A Onset-to-hospital: N/A Onset-to-needle: N/A
Wang, 2004 [47]	Video/ 75	12 (16%)	Mean age: N/A Female:N/A Median pre-NIHSS: 11.5 (Mean 14.3)	N/A	N/A	0	N/A	Home: 5 Rehab: 3 Nursing home: 1	Door-to-needle:104.9 Onset-to-hospital:70.9 Onset-to-needle:135.3
Wang, 2000 [55]	Telephone/ N/A	57	Mean age:71 Female: 40% Median pre NIHSS 14	N/A	5 (9%)	5 (9%)	6.2 days	Home: 31 Rehab: 14 Nursing home: 7	Door-to-needle: N/A Onset-to-hospital: N/A Onset-to-needle: 155
Wiborg, 2003 [42]	Video/ 153	2 (1.3%)	Mean age: 60 Female: 0% Median pre NIHSS: N/A	2	1 (50%)	N/A	N/A	N/A	Door-to-needle: 82.5 Onset-to-hospital: 45 Onset-to-needle: N/A

IV= intravenous, tPA= tissue plasminogen activator, N/A= not applicable, ICH= intracerebral hemorrhages, SC=Stroke Center

Different process indicators were analysed in the studies. Most studies reported time from onset of stroke symptoms to admission („onset-to-hospital"), time from admission to thrombolysis („door-to-needle") and time from onset of stroke symptoms to thrombolysis („onset-to-needle"). The mean "onset-to-hospital" time ranged from 54-70.9 minutes. The mean "door-to-needle" time ranged from 76-106 minutes and the mean "onset-to-needle" time ranged from 122-165 minutes. In the telephone based studies, length of stay varied from 4 days [54] to 12.3 days [49]. One telephone study reported a median length of stay of 5 days [51]. Of the VC interventions, one study reported a median length of hospital stay of 12 days [39] and in another study the mean length of stay was 11.4 days [49]. Just four studies reported on discharge destination. The majority of telethrombolysis treated patients were discharged home or to rehabilitation care.

The number of patients transported to a stroke center after telemedicine consultation varies in the studies. In Audebert et al. [40] 248 (13%) patients in the telemedicine group and 146 (13%) in the control group were transferred to other hospitals or departments. In Wang et al. [47] 75 patients were given consultations using telemedicine and 54 were transferred (72%) to a stroke center. In another study of 153 telestroke patients, 8 (5%) were transferred to a stroke center [42]. In one study fewer patients in the VC group were transported to the stroke center than in the telephone consulting group, 7 (9.1 %) and 13 (17.6 %) respectively [49]. One VC study reported that transfer was avoided in 11 cases [46]. Patients treated with tPA via telephone consultation were often transported to a stroke center for surveillance and monitoring [50, 51, 54]. In two VC/telestroke systems all tPA patients were transported to a stroke center [42, 45], although the total treatment number was very small (n=8). In two other VC studies 29 of 45 (64%) tPA-treated patients were transferred to a stroke center [43, 50].

5 Method and Material

5.1 Objectives and hypothesis

This thesis aims to explore if intravenous thrombolytic (tPA) therapy via a real time videoconferencing (VC) system followed by transfer to specialised stroke unit is safe and effective. A further aim is to evaluate the quality of care/service.

The hypothesis is that a VC based telestroke system can safely and effectively increase the use of intravenous thrombolysis in areas with insufficient neurological experience. After telethrombolysis the patients are transferred to a specialised stroke unit, which provides full coverage of guideline driven stroke care and the benefit of specialised stroke unit therapy. The specialised stroke unit also gives stroke patients access to new interventions, neurosurgery and neuroangiography interventions. A telestroke system may reduce inequalities in stroke care and also improve the quality of care in regional areas with lower levels of stroke care.

5.2 Research Questioning

Is intravenous thrombolysis delivery via VC system safe and effective?
Is the system of patient transport to a stroke unit following intravenous thrombolysis delivery via VC safe?

5.3 Study Design, Settings and Study Population

A retrospective controlled study was conducted to find an answer to these questions. The telemedicine group consisted of patients who were all treated with intravenous thrombolysis via VC between the years 2006-2009. In total there were five regional hospitals connected to a stroke unit via telemedicine (for more information please see chapter 4.4.4 Study Intervention). The control group consisted of patients who were treated with intravenous thrombolysis at a specialised stroke unit. Inclusion criteria: First time ischemic stoke patients of age 18 or older, treated with intravenous thrombolysis within 4.5 hours.

Exclusion criteria: previous stroke history, patients arriving 24 hours after stroke onset to the stroke unit, patients with severe disabilities (NIHSS score over 25 at admission).

5.4 Data Collection

For the data collection a list of different parameters and outcome measurements based on a systematic review of telemedicine in acute stroke care [36] was constructed (appendix 1). Data on the telemedicine group was mainly collected through the Austrian Stroke-Unit-Registry (Gesundheit Österreich GmbH), patients' journals and telestroke sheets. The control group was identified through the Austrian Stroke-Unit-Registry.

A telestroke sheet was used for each VC involving among others a criteria list for intravenous thrombolysis, patient name, date of birth, NIHSS and RS (Appendix 2). In the telemedicine group scores from the mRS before intravenous thrombolysis were missing (incomplete registration of telestroke sheets). These values were reconstructed by an experienced stroke neurologist analysing the patient journals.

Telestroke patients treated with thrombolysis were either identified through the telestroke sheets or through an admission registration book at the stroke unit. Every patient treated at the stroke unit was chronologically registered by name and with an individual patient number/ID in this book. Telestroke patients treated with intravenous thrombolysis were also documented in the admission registration book. With the patient number/ID it was possible to identify the patient in the hospital clinical information system (CIS) and in the Austrian Stroke-Unit-Registry in order to collect patient relevant information. Patient data was downloaded from the Austrian Stroke-Unit-Registry at 20.01.2010.

The Austrian Stroke-Unit-Registry has been administered since 2003 by the Gesundheit Österreich GmbH as an initiative from the Federal Government of Austrian [56]. In 2008 26 out of the 32 Austrian stroke units participated actively in the Austrian Stroke-Unit-Registry. The main objective of the registry is quality assurance and quality improvement of stroke-treatment in stroke units. The participating stroke units document their cases using a web-based database [57]. Data entry is online, anonymous and password secured. The register contains epidemiological, clinical, diagnostic and therapeutic data, as well as scores necessary for the compliance with the structure criteria. Follow up data are evaluated after three months. The participating centres have the ability to dispose of their own data.

5.5 Outcomes Measures

Main outcome measures:

For effectiveness: mortality, neurological status (in-/dependency) using NIHSS and mRS.
For safety: mortality, complications during transfer and complications during hospital stay.

Secondary outcome measures:
For analysing the quality of care/service the following measurements were used; length of stay, in-hospital complications, discharge destination, patient transport, patient admission (in academic hospital), processes of service (onset-to-needle and onset-to-stroke unit), medical treatments including PTA and secondary prophylaxis. At the 3 month follow-up, patient status, living situation and mRS were analysed.

Modified Rankin Scale (mRS)
The mRS is commonly used to measure disability after stroke. The 7-point scale (0-6) attempts to measure functional independence, incorporating the WHO components of body function, activity and participation (Appendix 3). The validity and reliability of the mRS in stroke outcomes have been well documented [58].

The National Institutes of Health stroke scale (NIHSS)
The NIHSS is a 15-item impairment scale which provides a quantitative measure of a standard neurological examination. Scores range from 0-42 points (appendix 4). Higher scores indicate greater impairment. The scale assesses level of consciousness, extraocular movements, visual fields, facial muscle function, extremity strength, sensory function, coordination (ataxia), language (aphasia), speech (dysarthria) and hemi-inattention (neglect). The NIHSS is an important tool for initial assessments of patients with stroke in emergency departments, hospitals or in the pre-hospital setting [59]. The NIHSS is a reliable and feasible tool in VC [60-62].

5.6 Statistical Analysis

Binary variables were analysed using a Chi^2-Test (Fisher´s Exact Test). Continuous variables (as age and time) were analysed with a T-Test (two-tailed). Descriptive statistics were used for the mRS (percentage allocation) a dichotomized analysis with Chi^2-Test (Fisher´s Exact Test) was also used for the mRS. Statistical analysis was performed with SPSS® Statistics18.0. The collected data was tested for correlations and plausibility according to Nonnemacher et al. [63].

5.7 Study Intervention: Telestroke in the county of Salzburg (TESSA)

TESSA is based on a high-quality videoconference system linking five regional hospitals with a stroke center/ specialised stroke unit (Tab. 4.7-2). The specialised stroke unit is a part of the clinic of neurology at the Christian-Doppler-Clinic, Salzburg, which is a leading research hospital in Salzburg. The regional hospitals are situated between 20 and 129 km from the specialised stroke unit.

Tab. 4.7-2: TESSA Cooperating hospitals

Hospital	Distances* (km) air/car	Neurological department	Technology	Transfer Megabit/second
Hallein	16/20	No	Phone and teleradiology	2
Schladming	68/93	No	VSX 7000	2
Schwarzach	55/70	Yes	VSX 7000	2
Tamsweg	96/129	No	VSX 7000	200
Zell am See	55/81	No	VSX 7000	2

*Calculation with google maps

Remote video-examination of patients was performed using a video-conferencing system. The system provides real time transmission of video and audio between the local hospital and the stroke center. Videoconferencing allowed the patient, the patient's family and both physicians to see and hear each other in full colour using two pan, tilt and zoom cameras connected to VGA televisions on each end. A VSX 7000 system (PolyCom, Inc.) was installed in the regional hospitals and a VSX 6000 system was installed in the specialised stroke unit. Physicians in the emergency departments initiated the consultation by calling the on call stoke neurologist in the stroke unit when a possible candidate for intravenous thrombolysis was identified. A specialized stroke team in the stroke unit provide 24h support to emergency physicians in the regional hospitals via the real time VC system. All patients were examined by a stroke neurologist who completed a NIHSS, reviewed tPA eligibility, viewed computed tomography (CT) scans of the head and provided recommendations on stroke management. All hospitals had the ability to send CT and/or MRI scans using a DICOM standard protocol (teleradiology). Data was transmitted at between 2 and 200 Megabit/second depending on hospital IP connectivity.

If a stroke patient was suitable for intravenous thrombolytic therapy the infusion was started during VC and could be continued during patient transport. During intravenous telethrombolysis the patients were transferred by either ambulance or helicopter to the stroke unit for further monitoring and surveillance. This system allows stroke patients in regional areas full availability to guideline driven stroke care including neurosurgery and neuroangiography interventions.

6 Results

434 stroke patients registered in the Austrian Stroke-Unit-Registry were treated with intravenous thrombolysis in the Christian-Doppler-Clinic, Salzburg between 2006 to 2009. Of those 35 Patients were treated via telemedicine (TESSA). 14 telestroke patients were identified through telestroke sheets or patient journals/admission books. In total 49 patients were treated with intravenous thrombolysis via telemedicine between 2006 and 2009. Two patients were excluded due to previous stroke history. 399 stroke patients were treated with intravenous thrombolysis between 2006 to 2009 at the specialised stroke unit. 304 remained as controls due to correlations and plausibility testing and inclusion/exclusion criteria. 70 patients were excluded due to previous stroke history. 12 patients were excluded due to severe impairment at admission (NIHSS>25). Two patients were excluded due to the age criteria (≥18 years). Six patients were treated with intravenous thrombolysis after 4.5 hours, by defining the penumbra in the MRI. One patient was excluded due to incomplete data and four patients were excluded because of arriving later than 24 hours after stroke onset at the stroke unit. Baseline characteristics are presented in table 5-3. Overall, no significant differences between the groups were found at baseline. The mean patient age was 66.5 years (SD ±14.4) in the telemedicine group and 71.0 years (SD ±15.5) in the control group. There were no significant differences between the telemedicine and the control group when comparing risk factors except for smokers. The telemedicine group included more smokers 32.4% versus 16.3% in the control group (p=0.032). A majority of the stroke patients had no or minor neurological disability before insult. This was explored using a dichotomized analysis (0-1) of the mRS. 93.6% of the patients in the telemedicine group compared to 87.2% in the control group (p=0.331) had good clinical function before stroke onset (p=0.475).

Tab. 5-3: Baseline data

	Telemedicine	Control	p-value
Number of patients included	47	304	
Excluded patients	2	95	
Age (mean/± SD)[median]	66.5 (±14.6) [72]	71.0 (±15.5) [74.5]	0.062^1
Sex (female, %)	16 (34%)	152 (50%)	
Comorbidities			
Diabetes mellitus	8 (17.4%) (n=46)	57 (19.3%) (n=296)	0.843^2
Hypertension	29 (63%) (n=46)	218 (72.9%) (n=299)	0.218^2
Myocardial infarction	2 (4.3%) (n=47)	23 (7.7%) (n=300)	0.552^2
Atrial fibrillation	17 (37.8%) (n=45)	107 (37.3%) (n=287)	1.000^2
Hypercholesteremia	21 (45.7%) (n=46)	135 (45.9%) (n=294)	1.000^2
Other cardiac disease	13 (27.7%) (n=47)	54 (18.4%) (n=294)	0.165^2
Peripheral arterial disease	0 (n=47)	10 (3.4%) (n=297)	0.369^2
Current alcohol use^3	1 (3.0 %) (n=33)	6 (2.2%) (n=268)	0.560^2
Current tobacco use	11 (32.4%) (n=34)	44 (16.3%) (n=270)	0.032^{2*}
Rankin scale prior stroke	(n=47)	(n=304)	
No or minor disability ^{4}	45 (95.7%)	278 (91.4%)	0.400^2
No or minor disability ^{5}	44 (93.6%)	265 (87.2%)	0.331^2

^{1} T-Test (two-tailed)
^{2} Fisher´s Exact Test (two-tailed)
^{3}(> 2/8 l wine or >1 bottle of beer (0.5l)/day or at least 5 days/Week), Chi-quadrate testing, T-test,
^{4} Dichotomized analysis, no or minor disability defined as a score of 0–2
^{5} Dichotomized analysis, no or minor disability defined as a score of 0–1
* Significant
SD= standard deviation

Performances of hospitals in predefined measures for quality of acute stroke care are shown in table 5-4. Mean length of stay was 6.4 (SD ±5.0) days in the telemedicine group versus 5.5 (SD ±4.6) days in the control group (p=0.255). In total 12 stroke patients died during hospitalization, 4 (8.9%) in the telemedicine group and 8 (2.6%) in the control group (p=0.056). The majority of the patients were discharged home, 14 (31.1%) in the telemedicine group compared to 79 (26.2%) in the control group. More patients in the control group (17.2%) were discharged to another department than patients treated in the telemedicine group (8.9%), but no statistical significance (p=0.195) was identified. More patients in the control group (20.5%) were discharged to a neurological acute care or intensive care unit compared to patients treated in the telemedicine group (6.7%) (p=0.024). In the telemedicine group 17 patients (37.8%) were transferred back to the consulting hospital.

Transport to the academic hospital (stroke unit) varied between the telemedicine and control group. Approximately 70% in the telemedicine group arrived at the stroke unit by ambulance with an emergency doctor present compared to 18% in the control group. Helicopter was used in 10 (25.6%) cases in the telemedicine group compared to 18 (5.1%) cases in the control group. Admission to hospital department varied between the groups. 34 (87.2%) patients from the telemedicine group were directly admitted to the stroke unit compared to 114 (37.5%) in the control group. The majority in the control group was admitted through the outpatient department (53.6%).

The mean onset-to-stroke unit time was longer in the telemedicine group 231 minutes (SD ±57.4) compared to the control group 108 minutes (SD ±71.9) (p=0.000). The mean onset-to-needle time was slightly shorter in the telemedicine group compared to control group but not statistical significant, 113 minutes (SD ±39.9) versus 122 minutes (SD ±47.2) (p=0.263).

Tab. 5-4: Indicators for quality of acute stroke care

	Telemedicine	Control	p-value
Length of stay in stroke unit. (days mean ± SD; median [95% -CI])	6.4 (±5.0); 5.0 [4.8-7.9] (n=43).	5.5 (±4.6); 4.5 [4.9-6.0] (n=304)	0.255[1]
Discharge destination:	(n=47)	(n=300)	
In hospital mortality	4 (8.9%)	8 (2.6%)	0.056[2]
Home	14 (31.1%)	79 (26.2%)	0.475[2]
Nursing home	0	6 (2.0%)	1.000[2]
Geriatric department or home for the elderly	2 (4.4%)	70 (23.2%)	0.003[2*]
Early rehabilitation	1 (2.2%)	25 (8.3%)	0.225[2]
Other department	4 (8.9%)	52 (17.2%)	0.195[2]
Neurological acute care bed or intensive care unit	3 (6.7%)	62 (20.5%)	0.024[2*]
Transfer back to consulting hospital	17 (37.8%)	N/A	
Patient transports	(n=39)	(n=260)	
Ambulance with emergency doctor	27 (69.2%)	62 (17.7%)	
Ambulance without emergency doctor	2 (5.1%)	170 (48.4%)	
Helicopter	10 (25.6%)	18 (5.1%)	
Private	N/A	10 (2.8%)	
Patient admission academic Hospital	(n=39)	(n=304)	
Outpatient department	1 (2.6%)	163 (53.6%)	
Specialty department	0	7 (2.3%)	
Direct to the stroke unit	34 (87.2%)	114 (37.5%)	
Emergency room	4 (10.3%)	20 (6.6%)	
Processes of tPA management:			
Onset to stroke unit (min.) mean (± SD) [95% -CI]	231 (±57.4) [214-249] (n=44)	108 (±71.9) [99-116] (n=280)	0.000*[1]
Onset to needle (min.) mean (± SD) [95% -CI]	113 (±39.9) [101-125] (n=42)	122 (±47.2) [116-127] (n=277)	0.263[1]

[1] T-Test (two-tailed)
[2] Fisher´s Exact Test (two-tailed)
* Significant
SD= Standard deviation
CI= confidential interval
N/A= not applicable

Cerebral oedema was the most common cause of death in both the telemedicine group and control group. 2 (50%) and 4 (50%) respective. Other causes of death registered were recurrent stroke and cardiac causes such as heart attack (tab. 5-5).

Tab. 5-5: Cause of death (in hospital)

	Telemedicine	Control
Cerebral oedema	2	4
Recurrent stroke	1	0
Heart attack	1	1
Other cardial cause	0	1
Other reason	0	2

After telethrombolysis all patients were transferred to a specialised stroke unit. According to the epicrisis no complications were reported during transportation. This indicates that it is safe to transport a patient after an intravenous thrombolysis from a regional hospital to a specialized stroke center.

In total five hospitals were connected to the specialised stroke unit. More than half of all consultations (51.1%) were initiated by one regional hospital. In total 96% of all consultations were initiated by three of the five hospitals (tab 5-6).

Tab. 5-6: Distribution of regional hospital s consultations

Hospital	Numbers of consultations
Hallein	1 (2.1%)
Schladming	9 (19.1%)
Schwarzach	1 (2.1%)
Tamsweg	12 (25.5%)
Zell am See	24 (51.1%)

Neurological examination was performed using NIHSS and mRS at different points in time (tab. 5-7). At hospital admission before intravenous thrombolysis the mean NIHSS was 9.9 (SD ±5.2) in the telemedicine group and 10.4 (SD ±5.9) in the control group (p=0.731). After intravenous thrombolysis and transfer to the specialised stroke unit the NIHSS in the telemedicine group was 9.1 (SD ±7.2). At discharge the mean NIHSS was 6.0 (SD ±7.3) in the telemedicine group compared to 6.8 (SD ±7.9) in the control group (p=0.500).

Percentile distribution of the mRS at admission, stroke unit discharge and the 3 month follow-up is presented in table 5-7. No differences were seen between the groups in mRS at admission using a dichotomized analysis (0-1) (p=0.231). More patients in the control group had a mRS of 1 or 2 at admission. At stroke unit discharge no significant differences between the groups in mRS were recorded. 38.3% in the telemedicine group had good functional outcomes at discharge compared to 32% in the control group (p=0.506)(dichotomized analysis 0-1).

The mRS at the 3 month follow-up showed no significant differences between the groups using a dichotomized analysis (0-1). In total 46.7% of the patients in the telemedicine group had good functional outcome at 3 months compared to 42.5% in the control group (p=0.694).

Tab. 5-7. Patients neurological function: NIHSS and Rankin Scale

	Telemedicine	Control	p-value
NIHSS (mean, ± SD [median])			
At admission[1]	9.9 (±5.2) [9.0] (n=19)	10.4 (±5.9) [10.0] (n=304)	0.731[2]
At stroke unit admission	9.1 (±7.2)(n=47)	.	
At stroke unit discharge	6.0 (±7.3) [4.0] (n=43)	6.8 (±7.9) [3.5] (n=292)	0.500[2]
Rankin Scale:			
At admission[1]	(n=47)	(n=304)	
0	0	1 (0.3%)	
1	0	13 (4.3%)	
2	1 (2.1%)	25 (8.2%)	
3	7 (14.9%)	41 (13.5%)	
4	24 (51.1%)	128 (42.1%)	
5	15 (31.9%)	96 (31.6%)	
Dichotomised 0-2[3]	1 (2.1%)	39 (12.8%)	0.027[4]*
Dichotomised 0-1[5]	0	14 (4.6%)	0.231[4]
At stroke unit discharge	(n=47)	(n=302)	
0	10 (21.3%)	61 (20.2%)	
1	8 (17.0%)	37 (12.3%)	
2	3 (6.4%)	26 8.6%)	
3	5 (10.6%)	37 (12.3%)	
4	6 (12.8%)	60 (19.9%)	
5	11 (23.4%)	73 (24.2%)	
6	4 (8.5%)	8 (2.6%)	
Dichotomised 0-2[3]	21 (44.7%)	124 (41.1%)	0.637[4]
Dichotomised 0-1[5]	18 (38.3%)	98 (32.%)	0.506[4]
At 3 months follow-up	(n=30)	(n=179)	
0	7 (23.3%)	37 (20.7%)	
1	7 (23.3%)	39 (21.8%)	
2	2 (6.7%)	17 (9.5%)	
3	2 (6.7%)	24 (13.4%)	
4	6 (20.0%)	24 (13.4%)	
5	1 (3.3%)	8 (4.5%)	
6	5 (16.7%)	30 (16.8%)	
Dichotomised 0-2[3]	16 (53.3%)	93 (52.0%)	0.842[4]
Dichotomised 0-1[5]	14 (46.7%)	76 (42.5%)	0.694[4]
Mortality during follow-up	5 (16.7%)	30 (16.0%)	

[1] Telemedicine group admission at the regional hospital and controls admission directly to the academic hospital (stroke unit).
[2] T-Test (two-tailed)
[3] Good functional outcome defined as a score of 0–2.
[4] Fisher´s Exact Test (two-tailed)
[5] Good functional outcome defined as a score of 0–1
* Significant
SD= Standard deviation

In-hospital complications were recorded as 11 (23.4%) patients in the telemedicine group compared to 66 (21.7%) patients in the control group (p=0.850). Reasons for complications are listed in table 5-8. The most common complications in the telemedicine group were progressive stroke and pneumonia, three cases for both (6.4%) In the controls haemorrhage bleeding was the most common in-hospital complication, 7.6% compared to 6.4% in the telemedicine group.

Tab. 5-8: In hospital complications

	Telemedicine (n=47)	Control (n=304)	p-value
Complications:	11 (23.4%)	66 (21.7%)	0.850[1]
Recurrent stroke	0	2 (0.7%)	.
Haemorrhage bleeding	3 (6.4%)	23 (7.6%)	.
Cerebral oedema	1 (2.1%)	5 (1.6%)	.
Cardiac arrhythmias	1 (2.1%)	3 (1.0%)	.
Cardiac decompensation	1 (2.1%)	2 (0.7%)	.
Sepsis	0	1 (0.3%)	.
Urinary tract infection	1 (2.1%)	8 (2.6%)	.
Pneumonia	3 (6.4%)	18 (5.9%)	.
Extra cerebral bleeding	0	1 (0.3%)	.
Deep vein thrombosis	0	1 (0.3%)	.
Progressive Stroke	3 (6.4%)	14 (4.6%)	.
Myocardial infarct	1 (2.1%)	4 (1.3%)	.

[1] Fisher´s Exact Test (two-tailed)

No statistical differences between the groups were seen in regards to continued medical treatment including medication, percutaneous transluminal angioplasty and secondary prophylaxis (tab 5-9). Intravenous tPA treated patients were commonly (>50%) given acetylsalicylic acid, subcutaneous injection heparin and secondary prophylaxis in terms of lipid-lowering agents and/or antihypertensive. Percutaneous transluminal angioplasty and clopidogrel was seldom used. Acetylsalicylic acid in combination with dipidolor and intravenous heparin was rarely used (less than 3%).

Tab. 5-9: Medical treatment, PTA and secondary prophylaxis

	Telemedicine	Control	p-value
ASA	28 (65.1%) (n=43)	197 (66.8%) (n=295)	0.863[1]
Clopidogrel	5 (13.2%) (n=38)	23 (7.8%) (n=295)	0.345[1]
ASA & DIP	0 (n=38)	3 (1.0%) (n=295)	1.000[1]
Heparin sc.	22 (55.0%) (n=40)	149 (50.5%) (n=295)	0.617[1]
Dicumarine	8 (21.1%) (n=38)	73 (24.7%) (n=295)	0.692[1]
Heparin IV.	1 (2.6%) (n=38)	2 (0.7%) (n=295)	0.306[1]
PTA (stent)	4 (10.5%) (n=38)	18 (6.1%) (n=295)	0.296[1]
Secondary prophylaxis:			
Lipid-lowering agent	18 (47.4%) (n=38)	116 (48.5%) (n=239)	1.000[1]
Antihypertensive	26 (68.4%) (n=38)	174 (72.8%) (n=239)	0.564[1]

[1] Fisher´s Exact Test (two-tailed)

ASA= acetylsalicylic acid, DIP= dipidolor, PTA= percutaneous transluminal angioplasty, IV=intravenous, sc= subcutaneous injection

In total complete follow-up data was obtained from 30 (63.8%) patients in the telemedicine group and from 188 (72.3%) patients in the control group. Respondents were not obtained in 13 (27.7%) cases in the telemedicine group versus 64 (24.6%) cases in the control group. Out of the controls, data was missing in 44 (14.5%) cases. At the 3 month follow-up five (16.7%) patients had died in the telemedicine group compared to 30 (16.0%) in the control group (p=1.000). The overall mortality was 19.1% (9/47) in the telemedicine group and 12.5% (38/304) in control group (p=0.248).

Most patients were living at home alone or with a family member/friend. In the telemedicine group 20% were living at home alone compared to 10.7% in the control group (p=0.190). 72% of the telemedicine group were living with a family member or friend versus 78.7% from the control group (p=0.445). 8% of the telemedicine group were living in a retirement home or caring home compared to 10.7% of the control group (p=1.000)(tab 5-10).

Tab. 5-10: Patient status and living situation at 3 months follow-up

	Telemedicine	**Control**	**p-value**
Drop outs (%)	13 (27.7%)	44 (14.5%)	
Carried out	30 (63.8%)	188 (72.3%)	0.294[1]
Patient or other respondent not attained	13 (27.7%)	64 (24.6%)	0.715[1]
In-hospital mortality	4 (8.5%)	8 (3.1%)	0.094[1]
Mortality during follow-up	5 (16.7%)	30 (16.0%)	1.000[1]
Overall mortality	9/47 (19.1%)	38/304 (12.5%)	0.248[1]
Living situation:	(n=25)	(n=150)	
At home alone	5 (20%)	16 (10.7%)	0.190[1]
At home with family member or friend	18 (72.0%)	118 (78.7%)	0.445[1]
Retirement home or care home	2 (8.0%)	16 (10.7%)	1.000[1]

[1] Fisher's Exact Test (two-tailed)

7 Discussion

Disparities in access to healthcare services exist due to geographical barriers and limited resources. Rural locations often lack the resources for adequate acute stroke care. The purpose of telestroke is to transfer knowledge and experience of stroke management into areas with insufficient neurological services. Telemedicine networks usually seek to establish connections between remote locations and provide specialist support through different types of videoconferencing and/or telephone systems. Most of these systems allow the transfer of radiology images (teleradiology) and clinical data.

The TESSA model aims to broaden the use of intravenous thrombolysis in areas with insufficient neurological presence. After telethrombolysis the patient was transported to a specialised stroke unit for surveillance and monitoring. This allows the patient full access to guideline driven stroke care including neurosurgery and neuroangiography interventions. Patients who receive organised stroke unit care and intravenous thrombolysis are more likely to survive and make a good recovery compared to patients treated in/on general medical wards [3]. An increase in the use of intravenous thrombolysis has also been reported as cost-effective in terms of quality adjusted life years (QALY) gained.

In terms of age and the NIHSS before treatment, the baseline characteristics of telethrombolysis populations identified in the literature were comparable to the TESSA study population. Age is an important predictor that influences health outcome after stroke. The in-hospital mortality in this study (8.9%) is hard to compare with other telethrombolysis studies where small study populations strongly influence the mortality rate. The mortality ranged from 0-50% in the telethrombolysis studies identified in the literature search [36]. Only two studies involved more than 100 telethrombolysis patients. In these studies the in-hospital mortality rates were 3.5% [41] and 10.4% [39], which is comparable to the mortality rate in this original work. The relatively high in-hospital mortality rate in the telemedicine group (8.9%) compared to the control group (2.6%) can partly be explained by the small number of patients in the telemedicine group (n=47).

Long term studies on telestroke have reported better health outcomes for patients treated in telestroke hospitals compared to conventional treated stroke patients. This includes reduced dependency and mortality at 6, 12 and 30 months follow-up [64]. Only two telethrombolysis studies reported on mortality and neurological clinical outcomes at 3 months follow-up [50, 65]. In one study the overall mortality rate at 3 months follow-up was 11.2% and 38.2% of the patients had good functional outcome (mRS dichotomized analysis, 0-1) [65]. In another telethrombolysis study with a small population the overall mortality rate in the VC group was 39% (n=12) and 30% (n=9) had good functional outcome (mRS dichotomized analysis, 0-1) compared to 12% (n=3) and 32% (n=8) in the telephone group [50]. These results are comparable to the 3 months follow-up results of the telemedicine group in this study. The overall mortality at 3 months follow-up was 19.1% and 46.7% of the patients had a good functional outcome (mRS dichotomized analysis, 0-1).

Comparing results from randomized clinical trials on intravenous thrombolysis with results from telethrombolysis studies is interesting and can give an indication of the safety of the telestroke intervention. The mortality rate and mRS at 3 months follow-up from clinical trials and telethrombolysis studies is presented in table 6-11. The mortality rate at 3 months follow-up in The National Institute of Neurological Disorders And Stroke rt-PA stroke study group (NINDS study) was 17%. A dichotomized analysis (0-1) of the mRS showed that 39% of the patients had a good functional outcome at 3 months follow-up [66]. In the Canadian Alteplase for Stroke Effectiveness Study (CASES) after 3 months the mortality rate was 22.3% and 36.8% of the patients had good functional outcome [67].

Tab. 6-11: Comparisons of safety of tPA treatment (3h window)

	TESSA	TEMPiS (telemedical group) [65]	Meyer [50] VC	TC	NINDS[66]	CASES [67]
Number of tPA-treated patients	47	170	31	25	312	1135
Median age (years)	72	71	N/A	N/A	67	73
Median NIHSS at admission	N/A	12	N/A	N/A	14	14
mRS (0-1) at 3 months (%)	46.7	38.2	30%	32%	39	36.8
Overall mortality at 3 months (%)	19.1	11.8	39%	12%	17	22.3

VC=Videoconferencing, TC= Telephone consulting, N/A= not applicable

Different outcome analysing processes of intravenous delivery were identified in the literature. The mean onset-to-needle time reported in the literature ranged from 122-165 minutes, which is slightly longer than the results from this study (mean 113 minutes). Possible explanations for this result may be an efficient patient transport system and good communication between health care personnel.

The median length of hospital stay (stroke unit) in the TESSA telemedicine group was 5 days. In other telestroke networks the median length of stay ranged from 5-12 days. Telestroke networks often indicate that patient transfers can be avoided when using the system. This is true, but a very large number of telethrombolysis treated patients, ranging from 61-100% were tranfered to a stroke center/stroke unit after therapy.

Factors for Good Telestroke Practice

A key factor in the success of telemedical interventions in acute care is the implementation of stroke protocols/sheets to aid the triaging of patients and the standardization of care. These protocols normally also include guidelines for intravenous thrombolysis (tPA) treatment. Stroke education, initial training, ongoing education for health personnel and a 24 hour service have also been reported as key factors in successful telestroke interventions [38-45, 47, 54]. Some studies reported shorter processing times after the program had been running for some time compared to the early stages of implementation [39, 43, 44].

Increased public awareness and better pre-hospital stroke management, achieved by continuous educational activities in the regional hospitals were proposed as the reason for the increased use of tPA [44]. This is important due to the fact that most stroke patients arrive after the 3 hour tPA treatment window. Better recognition of stroke symptoms and improved understanding of this time-sensitive illness may reduce the time to hospital admission. Centrally organized emergency inter-hospital transfers were reported as an important factor for success in some studies [39-41, 51]. Collaboration between remote emergency departments and stroke centers is probably the most important element of a successful telestroke program [51, 68]. Having an option of patient transfer after telethrombolysis to a stroke unit will also provide the patient with the benefit of specialised stroke unit care.

Future perspectives and research

Each telestroke program is unique in terms of personnel, resources, technology, the use of different health outcome measures and process management. Standardised outcome measures would allow increased harmonization, making it easier to compare programs and determine which factors ensure the success of such programs [7]. A set of outcome and prossess measurement indicators have been proposed in a systematic review on telemedicine in acute stroke [36]. To improve the documentation and data management of telestroke patients this data should be integrated in a quality registry. To improve the data management in TESSA it would be preferable to integrate the telestroke sheets electronically to the Austrian Stroke-Unit-Registry. This would make it easier for future analysis by physicians and researchers.

Few studies assessed the impact of telestroke on resource utilization and costs. An increased use of tPA treatment has potiential for cost reductions and cost-effectiveness [19, 20, 22, 23]. Authors of a telestroke network stated that this service is only cost-effective when screening tPA candidates via video consultation. Telemedicine networks require a substantial capital investment in equipment, education and technical support. Components of the costs of the development and maintenance of a telestroke network include the telemedicine equipment, information technology support, the necessary clinical and administrative personnel, personnel training and accreditation, and allowances for on-call coverage [65]. Further prospective controlled research studies are needed to explore the cost and cost-effectiveness of telestroke networks.

Prehospital stroke interventions such as improved communication and information technologies in emergency transport services may improve stroke care by reducing the time from stroke onset to hospital admission[69, 70], as this would increase the number of patients sutible for intravenous thrombolysis.

The development of a stroke care model with an integrated telemedicine system may be adapted in other regions or in other fields of medicine, for example dermatology, teledialysis etc. The technology could also be used in home-based health care, for example stroke rehabilitation [37]. Telemedicine technologies may further more provide better co-ordinated follow-up of patients in the fields of nursing and health care.

7.1 Methodological Discussion:

This study has several limitations. This study is a retrospective controlled study where the data is mainly collected from a stroke unit quality register. Retrospective studies are subject to recall bias and the risk of incomplete documentation. A stroke quality register intends to monitor the quality of stroke management with an aim of improving stroke care by providing comparative feedback data on processes and outcomes, but the register may be biased due to inaccurate or incomplete data [71]. It is important to consider that only stroke patients admitted to stroke units are registered in the quality register. In Austria large numbers of patients are treated in neurological wards or general medical wards and are therefore not registered in the stroke unit registry. The registration of stroke patients in the register is based on a voluntary commitment. Approximately 80-90% of all stroke patients treated in the specialised stroke unit are registered in the stroke unit registry. Unpublished data from the Swedish national Riks-Stroke register show that patients who die during stroke care are less frequently included in the Swedish register [72]. It is difficult to assess if this is the case in the Austrian Stroke-Unit-Registry.

The NIHSS score before intravenouse thrombolysis was only available in 40% of the cases and scores on the mRS were reconstructed by an experienced stroke neurologist using patient's journals. The validity and reliability of this method is questionable and is open for discussion. Inappropriate documentation and infrequent use of the telestroke sheet was the reason for this approach.

The drop out rate at 3 months follow-up was quite high, 27.7% in the telemedicine group compared to 14.5% in the control group. One reason for the high drop out rate can be explained by the date chosen for downloading data from the Austrian Stroke-Unit-Registry collection (20.01.2010). 3 month follow-up data was not available in patients treated between 20.10.2009 and 31.12.2010.

8 Conclusion

Telethrombolysis administartion via VC, followed by patient transport to a stroke unit is a safe and effective form of patient management. Patients treated with intravenous thrombolysis via VC had comparable health outcomes at hospital discharge and at 3 months follow-up compared to those treated with thrombolysis in a specialised stroke unit. The results presented in this thesis on mortality and mRS at admission and at 3 months follow-up after telethrombolysis are comparable to other telethrombolysis studies and clinical randomized trials on intravenous thrombolysis in stroke. The delivery of intravenous thrombolysis using telemedicine technologies based on VC is feasible and safe. Telemedicine systems can support regional areas with insufficient neurological experience in delivering intravenous thrombolysis thereby improving the quality of care and helping to decrease inherent inequalities between regions. The TESSA model provides stroke patients in regional settings with better access to intravenous thrombolysis and the added benefit of specialised stroke unit therapy.

Standardized measures to assess telestroke services would assist in the comparison between telestroke and standard care and would facilitate comparisons across telestroke studies. More research is needed to explore the long-term clinical and economic impact of telemedicine technologies in stroke management, so as to support policy makers in making informed decisions.

This study shows that telethrombolysis has become a realistic treatment option for community hospitals without significant prior neurological experience when a transfer to a specialized stroke center/unit is not practicable within the 3-hour time window.

9 References

[1] Lopez AD, Mathers CD, Ezzati M, Jamison DT, Murray CJ. Global and regional burden of disease and risk factors, 2001: systematic analysis of population health data. Lancet. 2006 May 27;367(9524):1747-57.

[2] Caro JJ. Huybrechts KF. Duchesne I. For the Stroke Economic Analysis Group. Management patterns and costs of acute ischemic stroke: an international study. Stroke. 2000;31:582–90.

[3] Organised inpatient (stroke unit) care for stroke. Stroke Unit Trialists' Collaboration. Cochrane database of systematic reviews (Online). 2000(2):CD000197.

[4] Wahlgren N, Ahmed N, Davalos A, Hacke W, Millan M, Muir K, et al. Thrombolysis with alteplase 3-4.5 h after acute ischaemic stroke (SITS-ISTR): an observational study. Lancet. 2008 Oct 11;372(9646):1303-9.

[5] Hacke W, Kaste M, Bluhmki E, Brozman M, Davalos A, Guidetti D, et al. Thrombolysis with alteplase 3 to 4.5 hours after acute ischemic stroke. The New England journal of medicine. 2008 Sep 25;359(13):1317-29.

[6] Wardlaw JM, Zoppo G, Yamaguchi T, Berge E. Thrombolysis for acute ischaemic stroke. Cochrane database of systematic reviews (Online). 2003(3):CD000213.

[7] Deshpande A, Khoja S, McKibbon A, Rizo C, Jadad AR. Telehealth for acute stroke management (Telestroke): systematic review of analytic studies and environmental scan of relevant initiatives. Ottawa: Canadian Agency for Drugs and Technologies in Health (CADTH) 2008.

[8] Rohkamm R. Color Atlas of Neurology. Stuttgart: Georg Thieme Verlag 2004.

[9] Candelise L, Gattinoni M, Bersano A, Micieli G, Sterzi R, Morabito A. Stroke-unit care for acute stroke patients: an observational follow-up study. Lancet. 2007 Jan 27;369(9558):299-305.

[10] Kjellstrom T, Norrving B, Shatchkute A. Helsingborg Declaration 2006 on European stroke strategies. Cerebrovascular diseases (Basel, Switzerland). 2007;23(2-3):231-41.

[11] Isaac SW. Access to Health Services In Encyclopedia of Public Health Ed. Breslow L. New York: Macmillan Reference, USA. 2002.

[12] Adams HP, Jr., Adams RJ, Brott T, del Zoppo GJ, Furlan A, Goldstein LB, et al. Guidelines for the early management of patients with ischemic stroke: A scientific statement from the Stroke Council of the American Stroke Association.[see comment]. Stroke. 2003 Apr;34(4):1056-83.

[13] Adams H, Adams R, Del Zoppo G, Goldstein LB. Guidelines for the early management of patients with ischemic stroke: 2005 guidelines update a scientific statement from the Stroke Council of the American Heart Association/American Stroke Association. Stroke. 2005 Apr;36(4):916-23.

[14] Adams HP, Jr., del Zoppo G, Alberts MJ, Bhatt DL, Brass L, Furlan A, et al. Guidelines for the early management of adults with ischemic stroke: a guideline from the American Heart Association/American Stroke Association Stroke Council, Clinical Cardiology Council, Cardiovascular Radiology and Intervention Council, and the Atherosclerotic Peripheral Vascular Disease and Quality of Care Outcomes in Research Interdisciplinary Working Groups: the American Academy of Neurology affirms the value of this guideline as an educational tool for neurologists. Stroke. 2007 May;38(5):1655-711.

[15] Olsen TS, Langhorne P, Diener HC, Hennerici M, Ferro J, Sivenius J, et al. European Stroke Initiative Recommendations for Stroke Management-update 2003. Cerebrovascular diseases (Basel, Switzerland). 2003;16(4):311-37.

[16] Albers GW, Olivot JM. Intravenous alteplase for ischaemic stroke. Lancet. 2007 Jan 27;369(9558):249-50.

[17] Wahlgren N, Ahmed N, Davalos A, Ford GA, Grond M, Hacke W, et al. Thrombolysis with alteplase for acute ischaemic stroke in the Safe Implementation of Thrombolysis in Stroke-Monitoring Study (SITS-MOST): an observational study. Lancet. 2007 Jan 27;369(9558):275-82.

[18] Hacke W, Donnan G, Fieschi C, Kaste M, von Kummer R, Broderick JP, et al. Association of outcome with early stroke treatment: pooled analysis of ATLANTIS, ECASS, and NINDS rt-PA stroke trials. Lancet. 2004 Mar 6;363(9411):768-74.

[19] Demaerschalk BM, Yip TR. Economic benefit of increasing utilization of intravenous tissue plasminogen activator for acute ischemic stroke in the United States. Stroke. 2005 Nov;36(11):2500-3.

[20] Sandercock P, Berge E, Dennis M, Forbes J, Hand P, Kwan J, et al. Cost-effectiveness of thrombolysis with recombinant tissue plasminogen activator for acute ischemic stroke assessed by a model based on UK NHS costs. Stroke. 2004 Jun;35(6):1490-7.

[21] Ehlers L, Muskens WM, Jensen LG, Kjolby M, Andersen G, Ehlers L, et al. National use of thrombolysis with alteplase for acute ischaemic stroke via telemedicine in Denmark: a model of budgetary impact and cost effectiveness. CNS drugs. 2008;22(1):73-81.

[22] Fagan SC, Morgenstern LB, Petitta A, Ward RE, Tilley BC, Marler JR, et al. Cost-effectiveness of tissue plasminogen activator for acute ischemic stroke. NINDS rt-PA Stroke Study Group. Neurology. 1998 Apr;50(4):883-90.

[23] Sinclair SE, Frighetto L, Loewen PS, Sunderji R, Teal P, Fagan SC, et al. Cost-Utility analysis of tissue plasminogen activator therapy for acute ischaemic stroke: a Canadian healthcare perspective. PharmacoEconomics. 2001;19(9):927-36.

[24] Österreichische Gesellschaft für Neurologie. Schlaganfall Krankheit, Beschwerden, Ursachen. [cited 26.04.2010]; Available from: http://www.oegn.at/patientenweb/index.php?page=Schlaganfall

[25] STATISTIK AUSTRIA. Gestorbene 2008 nach Todesursachen, Alter und Geschlecht. 2010 [cited 09.02.2010]; Available from: http://www.statistik.at/web_de/statistiken/gesundheit/todesursachen/todesursachen_im_ueberblick/index.html

[26] Jahrbuch der Gesundheitsstatistik, Statistik Austria. 2008 [cited 03.06.2010]; Available from: http://www.statistik.at/web_de/dynamic/statistiken/gesundheit/publikationen?id=4&webcat=4&nodeId=65&frag=3&listid=4

[27] Di Carlo A, Launer LJ, Breteler MM, Fratiglioni L, Lobo A, Martinez-Lage J, et al. Frequency of stroke in Europe: A collaborative study of population-based cohorts. ILSA Working Group and the Neurologic Diseases in the Elderly Research Group. Italian Longitudinal Study on Aging. Neurology. 2000;54(11 Suppl 5):S28-33.

[28] Haas M. Status Quo der Schlaganfallversorgung in Ö. zur Integrierten Versorgung Schlaganfall/Telestroke in Salzburg. 2007.

[29] Audebert H, Audebert H. Telestroke: effective networking. Lancet neurology. 2006 Mar;5(3):279-82.

[30] Fisher M, Fisher M. Developing and implementing future stroke therapies: the potential of telemedicine. Annals of Neurology. 2005 Nov;58(5):666-71.

[31] Perednia DA, Allen A. Telemedicine technology and clinical applications. Jama. 1995 Feb 8;273(6):483-8.

[32] American Telemedicine Association. Telemedicine Defined. [cited 03.11.2009]; Available from: http://www.americantelemed.org/i4a/pages/index.cfm?pageid=3333

[33] Grigsby J, Sanders JH. Telemedicine: where it is and where it's going. Annals of internal medicine. 1998 Jul 15;129(2):123-7.

[34] World Health Organisation. Information Technology in Support of Health Care. In: Department of Essential Health Technologies, ed. 2003.

[35] Levine SR, Gorman M. 'Telestroke': The application of telemedicine for stroke. 1999:464-9.

[36] Johansson T, Wild C. Telemedicine in acute stroke management: systematic review. International journal of technology assessment in health care. Apr;26(2):149-55.

[37] Johansson T & Wild C. Telemedicine in Stroke Management - systematic review. . HTA- Projektbericht 2009, No. 029. Ludwig Boltzman Institut Health Technology Assessment,.

[38] Waite K, Silver F, Jaigobin C, Black S, Lee L, Murray B, et al. Telestroke: a multi-site, emergency-based telemedicine service in Ontario. Journal of Telemedicine & Telecare. 2006;12(3):141-5.

[39] Audebert HJ, Kukla C, Clarmann von Claranau S, Kuhn J, Vatankhah B, Schenkel J, et al. Telemedicine for safe and extended use of thrombolysis in stroke: the Telemedic Pilot Project for Integrative Stroke Care (TEMPiS) in Bavaria. Stroke. 2005 Feb;36(2):287-91.

[40] Audebert HJ, Schenkel J, Heuschmann PU, Bogdahn U, Haberl RL, Telemedic Pilot Project for Integrative Stroke Care G, et al. Effects of the implementation of a telemedical stroke network: the Telemedic Pilot Project for Integrative Stroke Care (TEMPiS) in Bavaria, Germany.[see comment]. Lancet neurology. 2006 Sep;5(9):742-8.

[41] Audebert HJ, Kukla C, Vatankhah B, Gotzler B, Schenkel J, Hofer S, et al. Comparison of tissue plasminogen activator administration management between telestroke network hospitals and academic stroke centers: The telemedical pilot project for integrative stroke care in Bavaria/Germany. 2006:1822-7.

[42] Wiborg A, Widder B, Telemedicine in Stroke in Swabia P, Wiborg A, Widder B, Telemedicine in Stroke in Swabia P. Teleneurology to improve stroke care in rural areas: The Telemedicine in Stroke in Swabia (TESS) Project.[see comment]. Stroke. 2003 Dec;34(12):2951-6.

[43] Choi JY, Porche NA, Albright KC, Khaja AM, Ho VS, Grotta JC, et al. Using telemedicine to facilitate thrombolytic therapy for patients with acute stroke. Joint Commission Journal on Quality & Patient Safety. 2006 Apr;32(4):199-205.

[44] Hess DC, Wang S, Hamilton W, Lee S, Pardue C, Waller JL, et al. REACH: clinical feasibility of a rural telestroke network. Stroke. 2005 Sep;36(9):2018-20.

[45] LaMonte MP, Bahouth MN, Hu P, Pathan MY, Yarbrough KL, Gunawardane R, et al. Telemedicine for acute stroke: triumphs and pitfalls. Stroke. 2003 Mar;34(3):725-8.

[46] Schwamm LH, Rosenthal ES, Hirshberg A, Schaefer PW, Little EA, Kvedar JC, et al. Virtual TeleStroke support for the emergency department evaluation of acute stroke. Academic Emergency Medicine. 2004 Nov;11(11):1193-7.

[47] Wang S, Gross H, Lee SB, Pardue C, Waller J, Nichols FT, 3rd, et al. Remote evaluation of acute ischemic stroke in rural community hospitals in Georgia. Stroke. 2004 Jul;35(7):1763-8.

[48] Wong HT, Poon WS, Jacobs P, Goh KY, Leung CH, Lau FL, et al. The comparative impact of video consultation on emergency neurosurgical referrals. Neurosurgery. 2006 Sep;59(3):607-13; discussion -13.

[49] Handschu R, Scibor M, Willaczek B, Nuckel M, Heckmann JG, Asshoff D, et al. Telemedicine in acute stroke: remote video-examination compared to simple telephone consultation. Journal of Neurology. 2008 Nov;255(11):1792-7.

[50] Meyer BC, Raman R, Hemmen T, Obler R, Zivin JA, Rao R, et al. Efficacy of site-independent telemedicine in the STRokE DOC trial: a randomised, blinded, prospective study.[see comment]. Lancet neurology. 2008 Sep;7(9):787-95.

[51] Frey JL, Jahnke HK, Goslar PW, Partovi S, Flaster MS, Frey JL, et al. tPA by telephone: extending the benefits of a comprehensive stroke center. Neurology. 2005 Jan 11;64(1):154-6.

[52] Kuhle S, Mitchell L, Andrew M, Chan AK, Massicotte P, Adams M, et al. Urgent clinical challenges in children with ischemic stroke: analysis of 1065 patients from the 1-800-NOCLOTS pediatric stroke telephone consultation service.[see comment]. Stroke. 2006 Jan;37(1):116-22.

[53] Rymer MM, Thurtchley D, Summers D. Expanded modes of tissue plasminogen activator delivery in a comprehensive stroke center increases regional acute stroke interventions. Stroke. 2003 Jun;34(6):e58-60.

[54] Vaishnav AG, Pettigrew LC, Ryan S, Vaishnav AG, Pettigrew LC, Ryan S. Telephonic guidance of systemic thrombolysis in acute ischemic stroke: safety outcome in rural hospitals. Clinical Neurology & Neurosurgery. 2008 May;110(5):451-4.

[55] Wang DZ, Rose JA, Honings DS, Garwacki DJ, Milbrandt JC. Treating acute stroke patients with intravenous tPA. The OSF stroke network experience. Stroke. 2000 Jan;31(1):77-81.

[56] Bundesinstitut für Qualität im Gesundheitswesen. Stroke-Unit-Register. [cited 03.05.2010]; Available from: http://www.goeg.at/index.php?pid=arbeitsbereichedetail&ab=179&smark=stroke&noreplace=yes

[57] Hofer C, Kiechl S, Lang W. [The Austrian Stroke-Unit-Registry]. Wiener medizinische Wochenschrift (1946). 2008;158(15-16):411-7.

[58] Banks JL, Marotta CA. Outcomes validity and reliability of the modified Rankin scale: implications for stroke clinical trials: a literature review and synthesis. Stroke. 2007 Mar;38(3):1091-6.

[59] Kasner SE. Clinical interpretation and use of stroke scales. Lancet neurology. 2006;5:603-12.

[60] Shafqat S, Kvedar JC, Guanci MM, Chang Y, Schwamm LH, Shafqat S, et al. Role for telemedicine in acute stroke. Feasibility and reliability of remote administration of the NIH stroke scale. Stroke. 1999 Oct;30(10):2141-5.

[61] Wang S, Lee SB, Pardue C, Ramsingh D, Waller J, Gross H, et al. Remote evaluation of acute ischemic stroke: reliability of National Institutes of Health Stroke Scale via telestroke.[see comment]. Stroke. 2003 Oct;34(10):e188-91.

[62] Handschu R, Littmann R, Reulbach U, Gaul C, Heckmann JG, Neundorfer B, et al. Telemedicine in emergency evaluation of acute stroke: interrater agreement in remote video examination with a novel multimedia system. Stroke. 2003 Dec;34(12):2842-6.

[63] Nonnemacher M. Weiland D. Strausberg J. Datenqualität in der medizinischen Forschung. Leitline zum adaptiven Management von Datenqualität in Kohortenstudien und Registern. Berlin: MWV Medizinisch Wissenschaftliche Verlagsgesellschaft 2007.

[64] Audebert HJ, Schultes K, Tietz V, Heuschmann PU, Bogdahn U, Haberl RL, et al. Long-term effects of specialized stroke care with telemedicine support in community hospitals on behalf of the Telemedical Project for Integrative Stroke Care (TEMPiS). Stroke. 2009 Mar;40(3):902-8.

[65] Schwab S, Vatankhah B, Kukla C, Hauchwitz M, Bogdahn U, Furst A, et al. Long-term outcome after thrombolysis in telemedical stroke care.[see comment]. Neurology. 2007 Aug 28;69(9):898-903.

[66] The National Institute of Neurological Disorders and Stroke rt-PA Stroke Study Group. Tissue plasminogen activator for acute ischemic stroke. The National Institute of Neurological Disorders and Stroke rt-PA Stroke Study Group.[see comment]. New England Journal of Medicine. 1995 Dec 14;333(24):1581-7.

[67] Hill MD, Buchan AM. Thrombolysis for acute ischemic stroke: results of the Canadian Alteplase for Stroke Effectiveness Study. Cmaj. 2005 May 10;172(10):1307-12.

[68] Demaerschalk BM, Miley ML, Kiernan TE, Bobrow BJ, Corday DA, Wellik KE, et al. Stroke telemedicine. Mayo Clinic proceedings. 2009;84(1):53-64.

[69]   Ziegler V, Rashid A, Muller-Gorchs M, Kippnich U, Hiermann E, Kogerl C, et al. [Mobile computing systems in preclinical care of stroke. Results of the Stroke Angel initiative within the BMBF project PerCoMed]. Anaesthesist. 2008 Jul;57(7):677-85.

[70]   LaMonte MP, Xiao Y, Hu PF, Gagliano DM, Bahouth MN, Gunawardane RD, et al. Shortening time to stroke treatment using ambulance telemedicine: TeleBAT. J Stroke Cerebrovasc Dis. 2004 Jul-Aug;13(4):148-54.

[71]   Asplund K, Hulter Asberg K, Norrving B, Stegmayr B, Terent A, Wester PO. Riks-stroke - a Swedish national quality register for stroke care. Cerebrovascular diseases (Basel, Switzerland). 2003;15 Suppl 1:5-7.

[72]   Glader EL, Stegmayr B, Norrving B, Terent A, Hulter-Asberg K, Wester PO, et al. Sex differences in management and outcome after stroke: a Swedish national perspective. Stroke. 2003 Aug;34(8):1970-5.

Appendix 1: list of data collection/ outcome parameters

Baseline Data	Complications
Patient number/ID	Recurrent stroke
Birth date	Small relevant bleeding
Sex	Cerebral oedema
Date stroke onset	Epileptic seizure
Time stroke onset	Hydrocephalus
Consulting hospital	Cardiac arrhythmias
Date admission to stroke unit	Cardiac decompensation
Time admission to stroke unit	Pulmonary embolism
Transport art to the stroke unit	Sepsis
Intern transport	Urinary tract infection
	Pneumonia
Stroke Scales	Haemorrhage bleeding
Rankin scale:	Deep leg vein thrombosis
before stroke	Progressive stroke (worsening within 24h)
At intravenous thrombolysis	
stroke unit admission	Myocardial infarction
discharge, stroke unit	Complications during transports (epicrisis)
3 months follow-up	
NIHSS:	
At stroke unit admission	**Treatment & Prophylaxis**
At discharge, stroke unit	Acetylsalicylic acid (ASA)
	Clopidogrel
Risk factors	ASS & DIP
Hypertension	Heparin sc.
Diabetes mellitus	Dicumarine
History of stroke	Percutaneous transluminal angioplasty
Myocardial infarction	Carotid thrombo-endarterectomy
Hypercholesterolaemia	Heparin iv.
Atrial fibrillation	Lipid-lowering agent
Other cardiac disease	Antihypertensive
Peripheral arterial disease	

Nicotine Alcohol **Processes of Thrombolysis Delivery** Time intravenous thrombolysis Time, onset-to-stroke unit (min.) Time, onset-to-needle (min.)	**Discharge** Length of stay (stroke unit) Discharge date Discharge destination Cause of death **3 Months Follow-up** Patient status Cause of death Living situation Rankin scale

Appendix 2: stroke sheet for VC (in german)

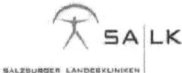

Checkliste Schlaganfall Telemedizin

1. **Patienten- ID**
   Name
   Vorname
   Geburtsdatum   Geschlecht
   Adresse
   Tel.

2.

		Tag	Monat	Jahr	Uhrzeit (24 h) auf Minuten
☐	Insultzeitpunkt	__ __	__ __	____	__ __ __ __
☐	Untersuchungszeitpunkt				__ __ __ __
☐	Intervall (Minuten)				__ __ __

   Ja/ nein   Vorderer Kreislauf
   Ja/ nein   Hinterer (Basilaris) Kreislauf
   ☐   rechts
   ☐   links
   ☐   bilateral

3. **Labor**
   Ja/ nein   Kontraindikation Lyse
              Laboruntersuchung (Minimum)
              BB
              Thrombo
              Elektrolyte
              PZ
              BZ
              GOT, GPT, GGT
              Alkal. Phosphatase
              Kreatinin

4. **RR (Grenze 185/110 unbehandelt)**   ___/___   ___/___   ___/___

5. **CT**
   Ja/ nein   Kontraindikation Lyse

              ☐   Media
              ☐   Basilaris

   Ja/ nein   Infarkt
   Ja/ nein   SAB
   Ja/ nein   ICH

6. **Indikation Lyse**

   Ja/ nein   auf Grund des Schweregrades gegeben

              ☐   NIHSS 5 oder weniger
              ☐   6- 25
              ☐   NIHSS > 25

7.

Ja/ nein	allgemeine Kontraindikation
Ja/ nein	Haemorrhagische Diathese
Ja/ nein	Manifeste oder relevante schwere Blutung
Ja/ nein	Vorgeschichte, vermutete oder manifeste SAB/ ICH
Ja/ nein	Vorgeschichte Schädigung ZNS (zB Aneurysma, intracer. oder spinale Chirurgie)
Ja/ nein	Hämorrhag. Retinopathie
	Vor 10 Tagen oder weniger
	☐ Herzmassage
	☐ Entbindung
	☐ Punkt. v. nicht kompressionsfäh. Gefäßen
Ja/ nein	Unkontrollierbarer, schwerer Hochdruck
Ja/ nein	Akute Pankreatitis
Ja/ nein	GI Ulcera während der letzten 3 Monate
Ja/ nein	Oesophagusvarizen
Ja/ nein	Arterielles Aneurysma, AVM
Ja/ nein	Tumor mit Blutungsrisiko
Ja/ nein	Schwere Lebererkrankung
Ja/ nein	Relevante Chirurgie oder signifikantes Trauma in den letzten 3 Monaten

8.

Ja/ nein	**Kontraindikationen im Kontext mit Insult**
Ja/ nein	Symptome länger als 3 Stunden
	unbekannter Beginn
Ja/ nein	Geringe neurolog. Symptomatik oder rasche Besserung
Ja/ nein	Schwere neurolog. Symptomatik (NIHSS > 25)
Ja/ nein	epileptischer Anfall
Ja/ nein	ICH im CT
Ja/ nein	SAB im CT nachgewiesen
Ja/ nein	Heparin i. d. letzten 48 Std. und eine TZ über Norm
Ja/ nein	Vorgeschichte Schlaganfall + Diabetes
Ja/ nein	Schlaganfall vor weniger als 3 Monaten
Ja/ nein	Thrombozyten unter 100 000
Ja/ nein	RR über 185 systolisch
Ja/ nein	110 diastolisch oder i.v. Behandlung
	(aggressiv) nötig
Ja/ nein	Blutzucker < 50> 400mg/ dl

9. Behandlungsbeginn

☐ Zell/ See
☐ Tamsweg
☐ Hallein
☐ Andere

☐ Körpergewicht geschätzt ____ kg
gemessen ____ kg

☐ Dosis Actilyse 0.9ml/kg
- 10% als Bolus i.v. über 1 Minute
- 90% als Infusion über 1 Stunde

☐ Gesamtdosis verwendet __ __ __ mg

10. Weiteres Vorgehen

Verlegung
- ☐ ja
- ☐ nein
- ☐ ischäm. Insult Lyse
- ☐ ischäm. Insult keine Lyse   - Intervall zu lange
  - Schweregrad
  - Kontraindikation
- ☐ ICH
- ☐ SAB

Verbleib in
- ☐ Zell/ See
- ☐ Tamsweg
- ☐ Hallein
- ☐ Andere

11. Vorgehen nach/ bei Verlegung

- ☐ Lyse syst. Media   3 h
- ☐ Lyse syst. Media   > 3h (zB ECASS 3)
- ☐ Lyse Basilaris systemisch

Intervention ischäm. Insult
- ☐ Media
- ☐ Basilaris
- ☐ Andere Gefäße
- ☐ Anderes Gefäß
- ☐ Methoden
- ☐ Topische Lyse
- ☐ Rekanalisation andere Methoden

Andere Maßnahmen ischäm. Insult
- ☐ Beobachtung
- ☐ Operation

Andere Maßnahmen ICH/ SAB
- ☐ Beobachtung
- ☐ Intervention
- ☐ Operation

Nach   1 Woche Rankin
       3 Mo

050404.telemedizin

Appendix 3: modified Rankin Scale

Modified Rankin Scale	At admission	Before insult	Discharge	3 months follow-up
0 = No symptoms	☐	☐	☐	☐
1 = No significant disability Despite symptoms able to perform all usual duties and activities	☐	☐	☐	☐
2 = Slight disability Unable to perform all previous activities but able to look after own affairs without assistance	☐	☐	☐	☐
3 = Moderate disability Requires some help, but able to walk without assistance	☐	☐	☐	☐
4 = Moderately severe disability Unable to walk without assistance and unable to attend to own bodily needs without assistance	☐	☐	☐	☐
5 = Severe disability Bedridden, incontinent, and requires constant nursing care and attention	☐	☐	☐	☐
6 = Dead	☐	☐	☐	☐

Appendix 4: National Institutes of Health Stroke Score (adapted from the Austrian stroke register, Österreichisches Bundesinstitut für Gesundheitswesen (ÖBIG)/Österreichischen Schlaganfall-Gesellschaft (ÖGSF)

NIH-Stroke Scale		Admission	Discharge
Level of consciousness	0 = Alert 1 = Not alert; but arousable by minor stimulation to obey 2 = Not alert; stuporous, lethargic or obtunded 3 = totally unresponsive (coma)		
Level of consciousness questions	0 = Answers both questions correctly 1 = Answers one question correctly 2 = Answers neither question correctly		
Level of consciousness commands	0 = Performs both tasks correctly 1 = Performs one task correctly 2 = Performs neither task correctly		
Best gaze	0 = Normal 1 = Partial gaze palsy 2 = Forced deviation, or total gaze paresis		
Visual	0 = No visual loss 1 = Partial hemianopia 2 = Complete hemianopia. 3 = Bilateral hemianopia		
Facial palsy	0 = Normal symmetrical movements 1 = Minor paralysis, flattened nasolabial fold, asymmetry on smiling 2 = Partial paralysis, total or near-total paralysis of lower face 3 = Complete paralysis		
Motor arm	0 = No drift for full 10 seconds 1 = Drift limb before full 10 seconds 2 = Drifts down to bed, but has some effort against gravity 3 = No effort against gravity; limb falls. 4 = No movement. Left Arm…… Right Arm……		
Motor leg	0 = No drift for full 10 seconds. 1 = Leg drift before full 10 seconds 2 = Leg drifts down to bed, but has some effort against gravity 3 = No effort against gravity; leg falls to bed immediately. 4 = No movement Left Leg…… Right Leg……		
Limb ataxia	0 = Absent 1 = Present in one limb 2 = Present in two limbs Left arm…… right arm…… Left leg…… right leg……		

Sensory	0 = Normal 1 = Mild-to-moderate sensory loss, but patient is aware of being touched. 2 = Severe to total sensory loss; patient is not aware of being touched		
Best language	0 = No aphasia, normal 1 = Mild-to-moderate aphasia; some obvious loss of fluency or facility of comprehension 2 = Severe aphasia; all communication is through fragmentary expression 3 = Mute, global aphasia		
Dysarthria	0 = Normal. 1 = Mild-to-moderate dysarthria; patient slurs at least some words and, at worst, can be understood with some difficulty. 2 = Severe dysarthria; patient's speech is so slurred as to be unintelligible in the absence of or out of proportion to any dysphasia, or is mute/anarthric.		
Extinction and Inattention	0 = No abnormality 1 = Visual, tactile, auditory, spatial, or personal inattention or extinction to bilateral simultaneous stimulation in one of the sensory modalities 2 = Profound hemi-inattention or extinction to more than one modality		
Total sum			

Danksagung:

Während des Studiums und der Erarbeitung der vorliegenden Doktorarbeit haben mich einige ganz besondere Menschen begleitet und unterstützt. Dafür möchte ich mich herzlich bedanken. Mein größter Dank gilt dabei meiner Freundin, Elisabeth Güntner, der ich für die wunderbaren, fachlich und hilfreichen Worte und Gespräche danke sowie für die große Portion Geduld. Auch der gegenseitige fachliche und methodische Austausch mit meinem Freund und ehemaligen Arbeitskollegen Stefan Mathis am Ludwig Boltzmann Institut Health Technology Assessment möchte ich herzlich bedanken. Die Leiterin des Ludwig Bolzmann Instituts Claudia Wild möchte ich für ihre Unterstützung danken. Meinem Betreuer, Herrn Prof. Gunter Ladurner, der mich beim Verfassen dieser Arbeit immer einen Schritt weiter gebracht hat und meine Freude am Thema stets aufs Neue entfachte, möchte ich ebenfalls herzlichen Dank sagen. Weiters möchte ich mich bei dem neurologischen Facharzt Dr. Sebastian Johannes Mutzenbach für seine fachliche Unterstützung bedanken. Und natürlich weiß ich vor allem die jahrelange Unterstützung meiner Eltern sehr zu schätzen, die mir das Studium ermöglicht haben.

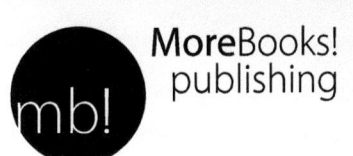

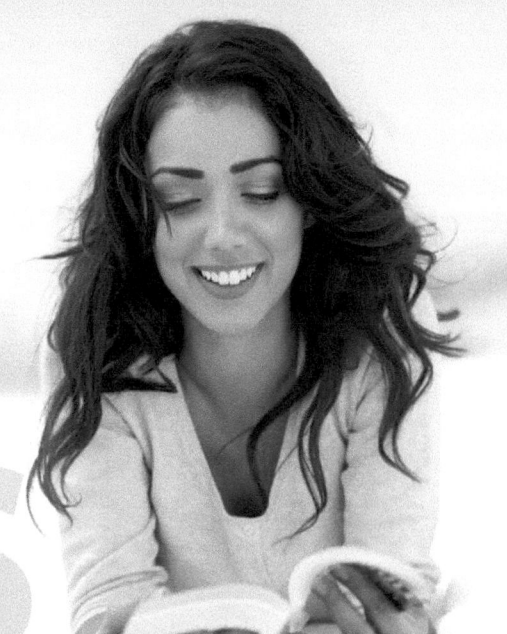

i want morebooks!

Buy your books fast and straightforward online - at one of world's fastest growing online book stores! Environmentally sound due to Print-on-Demand technologies.

Buy your books online at
www.get-morebooks.com

Kaufen Sie Ihre Bücher schnell und unkompliziert online – auf einer der am schnellsten wachsenden Buchhandelsplattformen weltweit! Dank Print-On-Demand umwelt- und ressourcenschonend produziert.

Bücher schneller online kaufen
www.morebooks.de

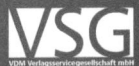

VDM Verlagsservicegesellschaft mbH
Heinrich-Böcking-Str. 6-8
D - 66121 Saarbrücken

Telefon: +49 681 3720 174
Telefax: +49 681 3720 1749

info@vdm-vsg.de
www.vdm-vsg.de

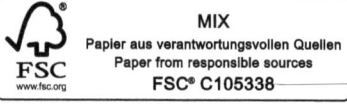

Printed by Books on Demand GmbH, Norderstedt / Germany